Transarterial Chemoembolization (TACE)

Pierleone Lucatelli
Editor

Transarterial Chemoembolization (TACE)

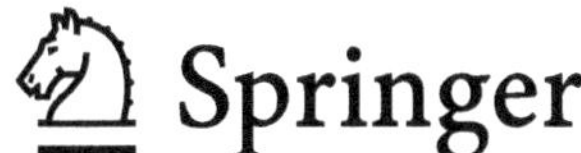

Editor
Pierleone Lucatelli
Vascular and Interventional Radiology
Azienda Ospedaliera Universitaria Policlinico Umberto I,
Sapienza University of Rome
ROMA, Roma, Italy

ISBN 978-3-031-36263-7 ISBN 978-3-031-36261-3 (eBook)
https://doi.org/10.1007/978-3-031-36261-3

This Springer imprint is published by the registered company Springer Nature Switzerland AG
The registered company address is: Gewerbestrasse 11, 6330 Cham, Switzerland

Foreword

Interventional Radiology (IR) has always been characterized by technical innovation. The expansive growth in devices and techniques has broadened the number of diseases amenable to treatment by minimally invasive means. In this context, embolization has become a major arm of current IR practice, with growing indications in diverse clinical scenarios. Its pivotal role has been widely accepted and recognized by surgeons and medical specialists.

In the field of hepatology, transarterial chemoembolization (TACE), which combines chemotherapy and embolization, is the standard treatment of BCLC stage B HCC, with a survival improvement compared to best supportive care, based upon a meta-analysis of five randomized clinical trials, and has therefore been included in international guidelines. TACE can also be used in BCLC stage A HCC patients when other treatments fail.

In modern oncology, the role of locoregional treatments to control tumor progression in liver-dominant disease has gained momentum. Transarterial treatments are always included in multidisciplinary team discussions for selected patients with cholangiocarcinoma and metastases from colorectal, neuroendocrine, and other primary neoplasms.

Over the past two decades, TACE has witnessed an increasing application because of a combination of the trend towards conservative treatments, advances in catheter technology, the introduction of new embolic agents, and refinements in digital imaging.

Improved discussion with clinicians and increased participation of IR specialists in multidisciplinary team discussions has further contributed to the worldwide applications of TACE. Procedure planning has become of paramount importance, backed by careful pre-procedural and intraprocedural imaging associated with 3D techniques, fusion imaging, and virtual reality.

The concepts and rationales vary for the different techniques; therefore, Interventional Specialists should use them appropriately, according to the patient's clinical conditions, tumor stage, and the clinical evidence of the treatment they are about to apply.

The development of this textbook has been triggered by the evolving medical and technical scenarios of interventional oncology, and by the perception that there was a need to take stock of the state-of-the-art of TACE.

The Editor of the book, Dr. Pierleone Lucatelli, from the University of Rome Sapienza, has put together a panel of internationally renowned experts, which will give the reader the big picture of TACE in the real world, together with a precise description of specific tools, techniques, and "how to" suggestions. This book also reviews the main indications of TACE, along with the imaging techniques used to evaluate the results of the embolization procedure and to address further treatment.

A comprehensive understanding of the rationale and practical knowledge of these techniques will be essential to IR specialists who are encouraged to use this book as a reference for the optimal and safe use of TACE in different clinical and anatomical scenarios.

University of Rome Sapienza
Rome, Italy

Prof Mario Bezzi,

Preface

Oncological Interventional Radiology, especially liver trans-catheter treatments, represents the focus of our hospital daily clinical practice and main interest in research.

The idea of this project was born after having completed the Cirse Standard of Practice on transarterial chemoembolization, which gave me the possibility to build a network among the bigger European high-volume centers involved in liver TACE.

Thanks to this opportunity we have raised together the idea that something technical in the field of interventional oncology, in specific of transarterial chemoembolization, was missing: that is why we are here commenting on this book.

This book presents the best knowledge about TACE, till 2023, with a wide panel of European experts presenting their best practice. The target audience is represented by all diagnostic and Interventional Radiologist involved in liver catheter-based treatments, with all levels of expertise ranging from resident, fellow, to expert operators. In fact, each chapter was intended to deliver to the reader the most technical consideration, in a step-by-step guidance fashion, as well as tips and tricks in order to start, or upgrade, their practice in liver embolization.

Rome, Italy Pierleone Lucatelli

Contents

1 Rationale, Definition, and History of Transarterial Chemoembolization

Bianca Rocco, Valentina Camelo, Valeria Feliciangeli, Carlo Catalano, and Pierleone Lucatelli

Transarterial chemoembolization (TACE) is a minimally invasive technique used for the treatment of liver's malignancies, mostly hepatocellular carcinoma (HCC). TACE allows administration of chemotherapy, carried in a mixture with Lipiodol (conventional TACE, C-TACE), or by drug-eluting beads (drug-eluting microsphere, DEM-TACE) [1], directly into the liver tumor's feeding vessels [2, 3]. TACE has been used in palliative treatments and unresectable HCC since the beginning of this century.

In 1929, the first vessel catheterization was performed by Werner Forssmann, a German surgeon, later described in his book *Experiments on Myself. Memoirs of a Surgeon*. Under local anesthesia, he catheterized—with a urethral catheter—his own antecubital vein and confirmed the tip of the catheter position in the right atrium with X-ray. In 1956, Werner Forssmann was awarded the Nobel Prize for Physiology or Medicine with André Cournand and Dickinson W. Richards [2].

Already in 1941, Farinas reported the first retrograde aortography by a urethral catheter passed up into the aorta through a trocar inserted in the exposed femoral artery [3]. Artery catheterization implied artery exposure, until in 1951, Pierce was the first to successfully attempt an aortography by percutaneous femoral artery catheterization, using a thin-walled polyethylene tube passing through a large-bore needle [4]. In these years, others started to employ a similar technique in order to catheterize the common carotid artery. The large-bore needle makes puncture difficult and limits its use to large arteries, also requiring larger holes than the catheter.

At Karolinska Sjukhuset, in April 1952, Dr. Sven-Ivar Seldinger (1921–1998), a Swedish radiologist from Mora Municipality, developed a safe and "simple" technique that allows safe access to the vascular system. The technique, later known as Seldinger Technique, permitted after percutaneous puncture to insert a catheter of the same size as the needle used into an artery [5] (Fig. 1.1). After this revolutionary development, endovascular techniques have evolved to treat several conditions affecting various organs.

B. Rocco · V. Camelo · V. Feliciangeli
C. Catalano · P. Lucatelli (✉)
Vascular and Interventional Radiology Unit, Department of Radiological, Oncological, and Anatomo-Pathological Sciences, Sapienza University of Rome, Rome, Italy

P. Lucatelli (ed.), *Transarterial Chemoembolization (TACE)*,
https://doi.org/10.1007/978-3-031-36261-3_1

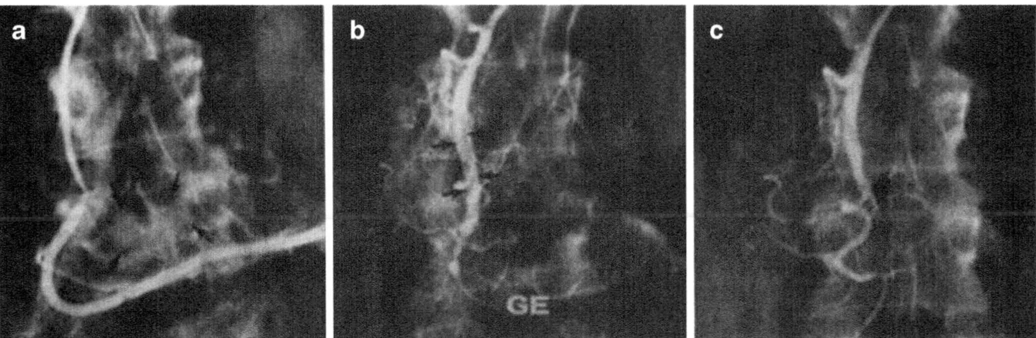

Fig. 1.1 Selective gastroepiploic (GE) and gastroduodenal arteriograms (Rösch J, Dotter CT, Brown MJ. Selective arterial embolization. A new method for control of acute gastrointestinal bleeding. Radiology. 1972 Feb). (**a**) Selective gastroepiploic arteriogram prior to epinephrine infusion shows extensive extravasation of contrast medium into the gastric antrum (arrows). (**b**) Selective gastroepiploic arteriogram after 20 min of epinephrine infusion and clot injection demonstrates extensive vasoconstriction of the gastroepiploic artery (GE). Blood clot forms filling defects around the catheter in the gastroduodenal artery (arrows). (**c**) Selective gastroduodenal arteriogram 14 h after clot injection. The gastroepiploic artery (arrow) is occluded, with good filling of the pancreatic branches

1.1 From 60 S to Late 70 S: From Diagnostic to Therapeutic Arteriography

Segmental catheterization of gastrointestinal arteries and radiological demonstration of bleeding were successfully reported in dogs in 1963 by Nusbaum et al. [6]. Therapeutic arterial embolization was first applied in the management of cerebral arteriovenous malformations through the use of tiny plastic pellets by Luessenhop et al. in 1965 [7]. In the early 1970s, arterial catheterization was used to arrest variceal bleeding in cirrhotic patients by arterial infusion of vasoconstrictors, like Pitressin, by Baum, Nusbaum, and Tumen [8–10]. Later, in 1972, Rosch applied transarterial embolization for the management of acute bleeding of gastrointestinal tract. The method consists in infusion of vasopressin, injection of autologous clot marked by tantalum powder so as to be fluoroscopically visible [11] (Fig. 1.1).

Several case series were published in those years about transarterial embolization through infusion of vasopressin or injection of autologous clot, silastic pellets, muscle and fat fragments, isobutyl 2-cyanoacrylate, silicone rubber, and Gelfoam or by mechanical occlusion by means of balloon catheters [12]. Katzen et al. in 1976 reported a case series of 19 patients treated with transarterial embolization (by injection of Gelfoam or autologous clot), of which 11 with bleeding of the upper gastrointestinal tract and 8 patients bleeding from other sites. Technical success was achieved in all cases and none of these patients had consequential hemorrhages.

The first tumors treated with embolization were renal carcinomas: In 1973, the first 19 patients were treated at the Karolinska Hospital in Stockholm by Almgard et al. [13] (Fig. 1.2). The embolization technique employed was the same already described 2 years earlier in an animal model by the same team: Muscle pieces were taken from the patients, finely minced and then suspended in a miscele of few milliliters of physiological saline and contrast medium into the renal artery, after renal artery catheterization. None of the patients experienced major complications and shrinkage of tumor was observed in all cases.

In the 70 s, preoperative angiographies were routine and the most accurate method of diagnosis of liver tumors, used as well to assess the resectability and curability of the lesions. Finally, in the late 70 s, angiographers were becoming

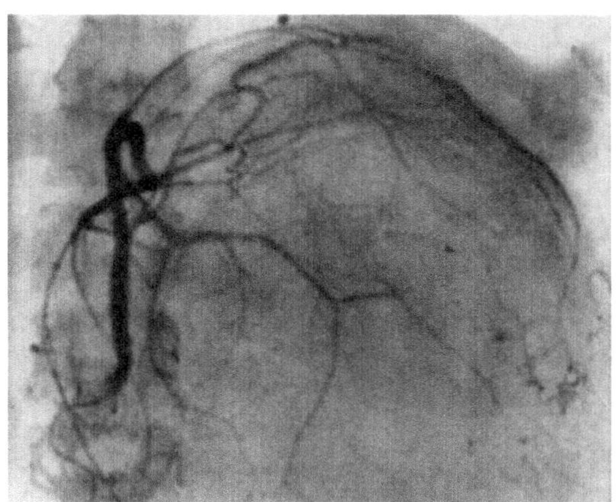

Fig. 1.2 Selective renal angiography showing a large tumor in the lower pole of the left kidney in an 83-y.o. man (Almgard LE, Fernstrom I, Ljungqvist A. Treatment of Renal Adenocarcinoma by Embolic Occlusion of the Renal Circulation. Vol. 45, British Journal of Urology. 1973)

more therapy-oriented and initial experiences in selective arterial liver embolization were described [14–17].

In 1973, Murray Lion et al. reported their experience in hepatic artery ligation for the treatment of 11 patients with liver secondary malignancies [18]. In six patients, also infusion of 5-fluorouracil in the portal vein was performed. None of the patients experienced liver failure, and many benefits, such as reduction of abdominal pain and weight gain, were achieved. Furthermore, liver biopsy performed after hepatic artery ligation demonstrated a reduction in the tumor size and extensive necrosis in the infused areas.

The fact that the hepatic artery occlusion is well tolerated was already known from the publication of Lucas et al. [19] published in 1971. Between January 1963 and February 1969, 119 patients with primary or secondary liver tumors were treated with infusion chemotherapy into the hepatic artery. Arterial access was obtained through a transbrachial catheterization, followed in 6–8 weeks by the permanent placement of a transabdominal catheter. The catheters were left in place for a very long and variable time, even more than 10 months. In 14 patients, complete hepatic artery occlusion occurred. However, the clinical course and hepatic function of these patients after the injection of the chemotherapeutic agents (5-fluorouracil or 5-fluorodeoxyuridine) were not altered by the occlusion of the hepatic artery.

Taking everything to account, the occlusion was well tolerated, concluding that the liver has a predominant blood supply from the portal system; also, the collateral arteries nearby protect it from parenchymal necrosis. For these reasons, the incidence of liver infarction is rare [20]. These results challenged the belief, established since 1933 by Graham and Cannell, that hepatic artery embolization with bloodstream interruption was lethal for patients and must be avoided [21].

In 1974, Doyon et al. reported the first French embolization of hepatic artery for the treatment of malignant liver tumors, using gelatin as the embolization agent [22]. In the early 80 s, Chuang and Wallace [23] described safety and oncological results of hepatic artery embolization performed (72 procedures in patients with liver malignancies, both primary and secondary). Three types of embolization were performed: peripheral embolization with Gelfoam, proximal using coils and combined proximal and peripheral with coils and Gelfoam. The majority of the patients experienced postembolization syndrome and median survival time was 11.5 months.

1.2 From Late 70 S: The Conventional TACE

First case series on embolization with drug and Gelfoam was published by Yamada et al. in 1977. The same group 6 years later reported their experience about 235 embolization procedures on 120 patients with unresectable hepatoma. The embolic materials employed and administered after catheterization of the branch of the hepatic artery that fed the tumor were gelatin sponge block cut into 1–2 mm pieces and permeated with an antineoplastic agent (10 mg of mitomycin C or 20 mg of Adriamycin) and contrast material (76% Urografin [meglumine and sodium diatrizoate]). In 75% of the cases, an objective tumor

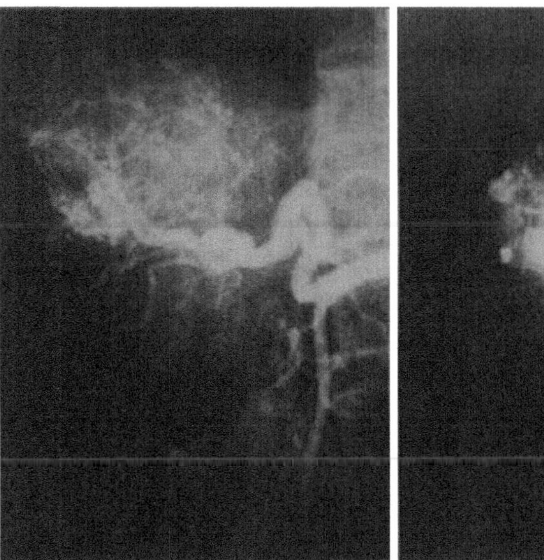

Fig. 1.3 Celiac angiogram of hepatoma before the injection of LUF (A, left) and plain film of the abdomen 2 months after the injection of LUF (B, right), showing retention of the contrast medium in the regressed tumor (Nakakuma K, Tashiro S, Hiraoka T, Uemura K, Konno T, Miyauchi Y, Yokoyama I. Studies on anticancer treatment with an oily anticancer drug injected into the ligated feeding hepatic artery for liver cancer. Cancer. 1983)

reduction greater than at least half was obtained (far better than the rate (6%) obtained with hepatic artery infusion for hepatoma) and 1-year survival rate was 44% [24].

Nakakuma et al. [25] were the first to report a selective and long-lasting retention of Lipiodol by the tumor in 1983. The team reported their experimental study on 77 rabbits and 6 adult patients with nonresectable liver cancer. The lobar hepatic artery where the tumor was located was ligated and then injected with Lipiodol Ultra Fluid (LUF). The oily contrast medium was found in all the branches of the injected artery. The X-ray films obtained immediately after detected the LUF in the vessels of the tumor and in the vessels of the normal parenchyma as well. After the third postoperative day to the seventh, the contrast gradually disappeared from the non-tumoral areas of the liver but remained focused in the cancerous portions. LUF was observed in the tumor tissue until 16 months after the injection (Fig. 1.3).

At that time, drugs employed by intra-arterial infusion for the treatment of HCC were 5-fluorouracil, Adriamycin, and mitomycin C separated or in combinations [26, 27]. Hirose et al. demonstrated that one administration of one of these chemotherapeutic by intra-arterial infusion, was superior to any method of repeated systemic administration [28]. These agents (Lipiodol and CHT) were consequently used in combination in transarterial therapies for HCC.

The name transcatheter arterial chemoembolization was used for the first time in the 80 s.

1.3 From the 80 S: Degradable Starch Microsphere TACE

In 1982, Dakhil [29] published a pilot study about the intra-arterial administration of starch microspheres (40 μm in diameter), rapidly degraded by serum amylase, to five patients with primary and metastatic liver cancer. Authors determined that arterial blood flow through the liver could be temporarily blocked, enhancing regional uptake and catabolism and decreasing systemic exposure to simultaneously administered hepatic arterial bischlorethylnitrosourea (BCNU).

Wollner et al. [30] in 1986 reported the results of a phase II trial about primary and metastatic liver cancer treated with hepatic arterial mitomycin C admixed with degradable starch microspheres (DSM). The oncological outcomes in those six patients were promising. A high response rate was achieved also by Carr et al. [31] in 1997, in the treatment of HCC with DSM TACE with doxorubicin and cisplatin in the treatment of HCC.

Later in the years, a deeper understanding of tumor growth mechanism gave doubt about carcinogenesis and ischemic potential of c-TACE. In fact, Xin Li et al. displayed that TACE, by interrupting blood flow to the tumor, induces necrosis but at the same time may create conditions that permit or even encourage angiogenesis and the reconstruction of blood supply of residual cancer tissue [32]. These lead to a reevaluation of degradable starch microsphere TACE, until its inclusion in CIRSE standards of practice on hepatic transarterial embolization [33].

1.4 The 90 S–2000: Evidences on TACE

In the 90 s, a lively debate was made about the utility of chemoembolization in regard to overall survival. The French Group for study and treatment for HCC published in 1995 [34] the results of a randomized trial where patients were randomly assigned to receive either Lipiodol chemoembolization (70 mg of cisplatin, 10 ml of lipiodol, and gelatin sponge [Gelfoam] particles delivered through the hepatic artery) or conservative management, involving treatment of complications and pain. The study was stopped after a sequential analysis showed the lack of the expected benefit from chemoembolization. Until the early 2000s, when a systematic review of randomized trials by Llovet et al. [35] was published, TACE had a limited role in the management of HCC. Llovet et al. in fact performed a meta-analysis including 7 trials (545 patients) of patients undergoing TACE and 7 trials (898 patients) treated with tamoxifen. Primary endpoints were overall survival and treatment response. Arterial embolization improved 2-year survival (odds ratio [OR], 0.53; 95% confidence interval [CI], 0.32–0.89; $P = 0.017$). Sensitivity analysis showed a significant benefit of chemoembolization (OR, 0.42; 95% CI, 0.20–0.88) but none with embolization alone (OR, 0.59; 95% CI, 0.29–1.20). Overall, treatment induced objective responses in 35% of patients (range, 16%–61%), while tamoxifen showed no antitumoral effect and no survival benefits (OR, 0.64; 95% CI, 0.36–1.13; $P = 0.13$). This study finally set the grounds for TACE's inclusion in several guidelines.

1.5 From Early 2000: Drug-Eluting Beads TACE

At the beginning of 2000, a novel embolization drug delivery system was proposed: the DC Bead (Biocompatibles UK Ltd.), a biocompatible, non-resorbable hydrogel beads that can be loaded with anthracycline's derivatives such as doxorubicin [36].

In preclinical studies, Drug-Eluting Beads TACE (DEB-TACE) demonstrates a high tumor concentration of doxorubicin, avoiding its significant passage into the systemic circulation with consequent less systemic toxicity. In fact, Lewis et al. [37] in 2006 reported the pathologic and pharmacokinetic findings from hepatic embolization in a porcine model comparing doxorubicin-eluting beads with bland embolization. Hepatic embolization with DC Beads demonstrated to be safe and well tolerated, with locoregional delivery of doxorubicin causing targeted tissue damage with minimal systemic impact. Similar results were obtained in the same year by Hong et al. [38] in a rabbit model.

In 2007, Varela et al. [39] confirmed in the first clinical experience the findings demonstrated in the preclinical studies. In this study, Llovet group demonstrated the same efficacy of c-TACE and DEB-TACE, showing at the same time that DEB-TACE prolongs the contact time between the cancer cells and the cytotoxic drug and reduces the concentration of chemotherapeutic in the serum (Fig. 1.4), potentially avoiding the onset of minor systemic effects like hematological toxicity, alopecia, mucositis, and skin discoloration.

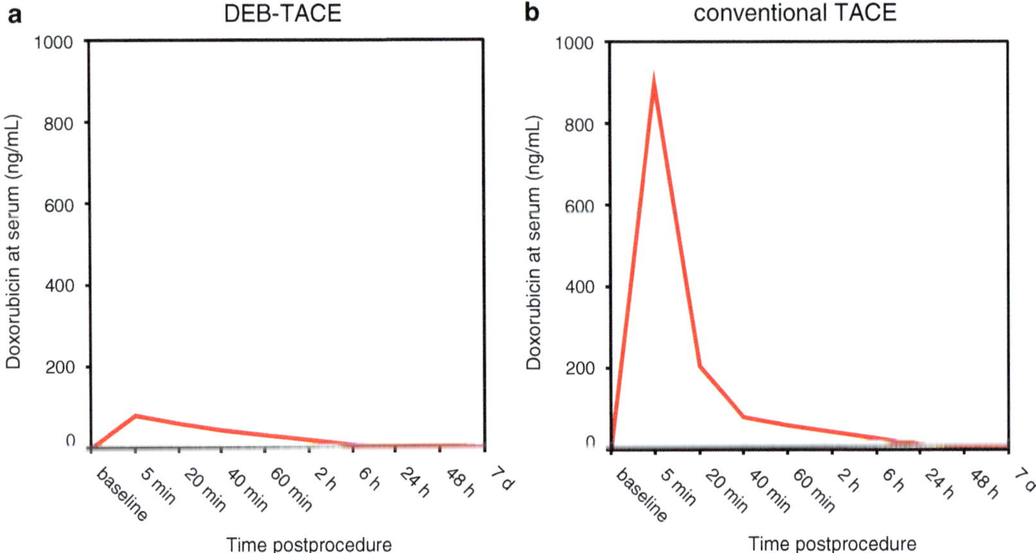

Fig. 1.4 Measurements of serum doxorubicin levels at different time points and AUC in DEB-TACE patients (**a**) and in the conventional TACE group (**b**). The AUC of group DEB-TACE is significantly lower than that observed in the conventional TACE, although the dose of doxorubicin was significantly higher in the DEB-TACE group. (Varela M, Real MI, Burrel M, Forner A, Sala M, Brunet M, et al. Chemoembolization of hepatocellular carcinoma with drug eluting beads: Efficacy and doxorubicin pharmacokinetics. Journal of Hepatology. 2007)

The Poon et al. [40] phase I/II trial published in 2007 also confirmed a low peak plasma doxorubicin concentration and no systemic toxicity.

Malgari et al. [41] in the same year reported the efficacy of DEB-TACE in 42 patients with confirmed HCC. Patients underwent superselective DEB-TACE every 2 months, until cessation of flow was achieved. CT revealed complete response in 65% and localized residual enhancement in 40% of cases. Also, in this study, disorders of hepatic function were not observed post procedure, while a substantial reduction in fetoprotein levels was observed.

Drug-eluting beads were also used in metastasis treatment. In 2008, de Baere et al. [42] reported their experience in the DEB-TACE for gastropancreatic endocrine hepatic metastases in 20 patients.

In another study of 2009 by Lammer et al. [43], it was displayed that there wasn't a statistically significant response rate, following the EASL criteria, in the TACE with loaded microspheres group, compared to the Lipiodol TACE group ($p = 0.11$), but it has once again been confirmed that there was a significantly lower toxicity of doxorubicin in the TACE with loaded microspheres group because of its lower serum concentration ($p = 0.0001$). In addition, it has been proved that DEB-TACE offers a benefit to patients with more advanced disease.

1.6 From 2008 to Nowadays

Irie et al. in 2008 employed a micro-balloon microcatheter in order to optimize TACE oncological performance, setting the ground for a new TACE technique: the balloon-occluded TACE (B-TACE). In fact, better Lipiodol deposition was allowed by inflating the micro-balloon, as it prevents proximal migration and leakage of embolization materials [44] as well as opens intrahepatic shunts that direct the arterial flow toward the tumor.

In 2019, Lucatelli et al. [45] described the efficacy and safety of B-TACE performed with polyethylene glycol epirubicin-loaded drug-eluting embolics in HCC patients. As mentioned previ-

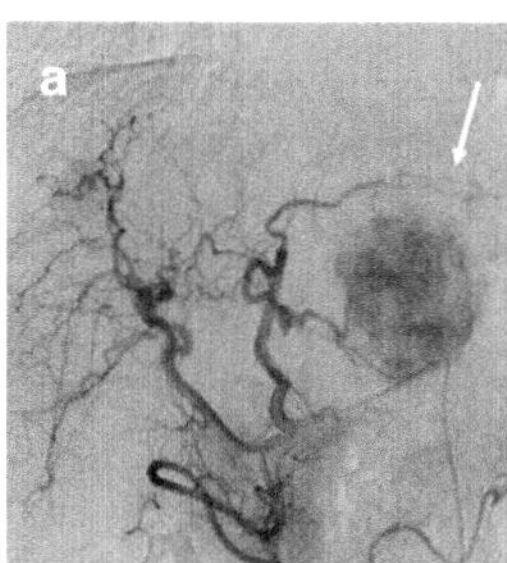

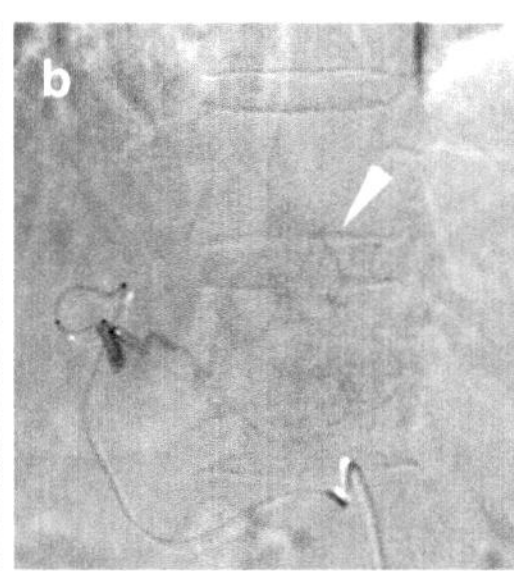

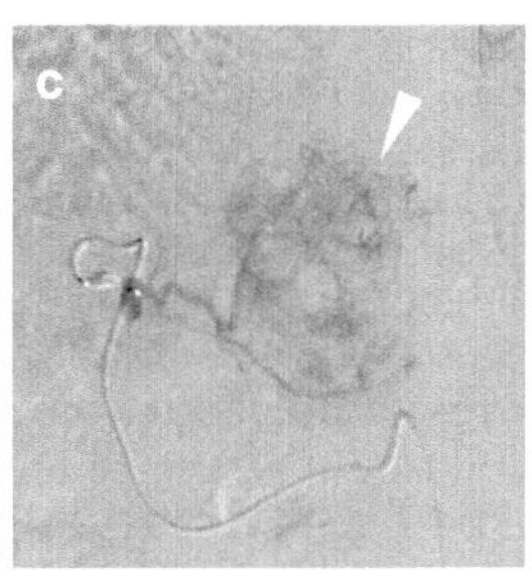

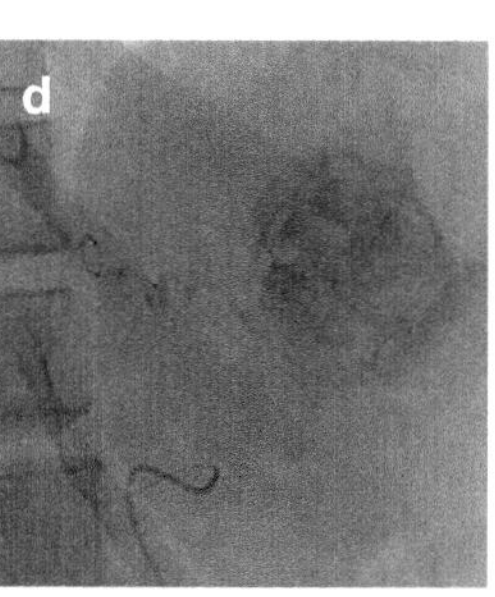

Fig. 1.5 A 56-year-old male with a single nodule of HCC with maximal diameter of 76 mm at II/III hepatic segments. Digital subtraction angiography (DSA) performed from the common hepatic artery (**a**) shows the hypervascular structure of the HCC in the left lobe (arrow). Superselective DSA of the tumor with deflated balloon (**b**) and inflated balloon (**c**) (arrowhead); single fluoroscopy image after the embolization (**d**) (Lucatelli P, Ginnani Corradini L, de Rubeis G, Rocco B, Basilico F, Cannavale A, et al. Balloon-Occluded Transcatheter Arterial Chemoembolization (b-TACE) for Hepatocellular Carcinoma Performed with Polyethylene-Glycol Epirubicin-Loaded Drug-Eluting Embolics: Safety and Preliminary Results. CardioVascular and Interventional Radiology. 2019)

ously, conventional TACE (c-TACE) has shown several limitations (procedure standardization, toxicity profile, pain), overcame by the introduction of drug-eluting microsphere transarterial chemoembolization (DEM-TACE). In this study, the efficacy of the combination of DEM-TACE with B-TACE was studied and it was proved that it is a safe procedure, associated with a high overall tumor response (Fig. 1.5).

Taking everything into account, it could be stated that TACE is a relatively new noninvasive technique that can be used for the treatment of liver malignancies, primaries and secondary, in order to increase overall survival. In the later years, several studies were made in order to improve its efficacy and reduce the side effects, as well as to enlarge the therapeutic field. Taking advantage of the intratumoral inflammation created by TACE with consequent expression of antigens usually hidden in the tumoral microenvironment [42], frontiers are open to combined treatment with targeted immunotherapeutic drugs.

References

1. Kudo M. The 2008 Okuda lecture: management of hepatocellular carcinoma: from surveillance to molecular targeted therapy. Vol. 25, Journal of gastroenterology and hepatology (Australia). J Gastroenterol Hepatol. 2010;25:439–52.
2. Werner Forssmann–Biographical. NobelPrize.org. Nobel prize outreach AB 2022. Sun. 22 May 2022. https://www.nobelprize.org/prizes/medicine/1956/forssmann/biographical/
3. Farinas LP. A new technique for the arteriographic examination of the abdominal aorta and its branches. Am J Roentgenol. 1941;
4. Peirce EC. Percutaneous femoral artery catheterization in man with special reference to aortography. Surg Gynaecol Obstet. 1951;133:544.
5. Seldinger SI. Catheter replacement of the needle in percutaneous arteriography: a new technique. Acta Radiol. 1953 May 1;39(5):368–76.
6. Nusbaum M, Baum S. Radiographic demonstration of unknown sites of gastrointestinal bleeding. Surg Forum. 1963;14:374–5.
7. Luessenhop AJ, Kachmann R Jr, Shevlin W, Ferrero AA. Clinical evaluation of artificial embolization in the management of large cerebral arteriovenous malformations. J Neurosurg. 1965;23(4):400–17.
8. Nusbaum M, Baum S, Blakemore WS, Finklstein A. Demonstration of intra-abdominal bleeding by selective arteriography. Visualization of celiac and superior mesenteric arteries. JAMA. 1965 Feb 1;191:389–90. https://doi.org/10.1001/jama.1965.03080050035009.
9. Nusbaum M, Baum S, Blakemore WS. Clinical experience with the diagnosis and management of gastrointestinal hemorrhage by selective mesenteric catheterization. Ann Surg. 1969;170:506–14.
10. Baum S, Nusbaum M. The control of gastrointestinal hemorrhage by selective mesenteric arterial infusion of vasopressin 1 diagnostic radiology. Radiology. 1971;98:497.
11. Rösch J, Dotter CT, Brown MJ. Selective arterial embolization. A new method for control of acute gastrointestinal bleeding. Radiology. 1972 Feb;102(2):303–6. https://doi.org/10.1148/102.2.303.

12. Doppman JL, di Chiro G, Ommaya AK. Percutaneous embolization of spinal cord arteriovenous malformations.
13. Almgard LE, Fernstrom I, Ljungqvist A. Treatment of renal adenocarcinoma by embolic occlusion of the renal circulation. Br J Urol. 1973;45:474.
14. Goldstein HM, Wallace S, Anderson JH, Bree RL, Gianturco C. Transcatheter occlusion of abdominal tumors 1.
15. Wheeler PG, Melia W, Dubbins P, Jones B, Nunnerley H, Johnson P, et al. Non-operative arterial embolisation in primary liver tumours, vol. 28. Br Med J; 1979. p. 242.
16. Yamada R, Nakatsuka H, Nakamura K, et al. Transcatheter arterial embolization therapy in unresectable hepatomas-experience in 15 cases. Acta Hepatologica Japonica (Tokyo). 1979;20:595.
17. Reuter SR. The current status of angiography in the evaluation of cancer patients. Cancer. 1976;37:532–41.
18. Murray-Lyon IM. Treatment of hepatic tumours by ligation of the hepatic artery and infusion of cytotoxic drugs. J R Coll Surg Edinb. 1972;17:156–61.
19. Lucas RJ, Tumacder O, Wilson GS. Hepatic artery occlusion following hepatic artery catheterization. Ann Surg. 1971;173:238–43.
20. Cleveland JC. Inadvertent interruption of hepatic arterial flow.
21. Roscoe Graham BR, Cannell D. Accidental ligation of the hepatic artery. report of one case, with a review of the cases in the literature.
22. Doyon D, Mouzon A, Jourde AM, Regensberg C, Frileux C. Hepatic, arterial embolization in patients with malignant liver tumours. Ann Radiol. 1974;17:593–603.
23. Chuang VP, Wallace S. Hepatic artery embolization in the treatment of hepatic neoplasms 1.
24. Yamada R, Sato M, Kawabata M, Nakatsuka H, Nakamura K, Takashima S. Interventional radiology hepatic artery embolization in 120.
25. Nakakuma K, Tashiro S, Hiraoka T, Uemura K, Konno T, Miyauchi Y, Yokoyama I. Studies on anticancer treatment with an oily anticancer drug injected into the ligated feeding hepatic artery for liver cancer. Cancer. 1983 Dec 15;52(12):2193–200. https://doi.org/10.1002/1097-0142(19831215)52:12<2193::aid-cncr2820521203>3.0.co;2-r.
26. Friedman MA, Volberding PA, Cassidy MJ. Therapy for hepatocellular cancer with intrahepatic arterial Adriamycin and 5-fluorouracil combined with whole-liver irradiadiation: a northern California oncology group study. Cancer Treat Rep. 1979;63:1885–8.
27. Misra NC, Jaiswal MSD, Singh RV, Das B. Intrahepatic arterial infusion of combination of mitomycin C and 5 fluorouracil in treatment of primary and metastatic liver carcinoma. Cancer. 1977;39:1425–9.
28. Hirose H, Aoyama M, Oshima K, et al. Chemotherapy of hepatocellular carcinoma–with special reference to one-shot intra-arterial infusion of a high dose of adriamycin. Gan To Kagaku Ryoho. 1982;9:2216–21.
29. Dakhil S, Ensminger W, Cho K, John Niederhuber Md, Doan KR, Wheeler R, et al. Improved regional selectivity of hepatic arterial bcnu with degradable microspheres.
30. Wollner IS, Walker-Andrews SC, Smith JE, Ensminger WD. Phase II study of hepatic arterial degradable starch microspheres and Mitomycin. Cancer Drug Deliv. 1986;3:279.
31. Carr BI, Zajko A, Bron K, Orons P, Sammon J, Baron R. Phase II study of Spherex (degradable starch microspheres) injected into the hepatic artery in conjunction with doxorubicin and cisplatin in the treatment of advanced-stage hepatocellular carcinoma: interim analysis. Semin Oncol. 1997;24(2 Suppl 6):S6-97–9.
32. Li X, Feng G-S, Zheng C-S, Zhuo C-K, Liu X. Influence of transarterial chemoembolization on angiogenesis and expression of vascular endothelial growth factor and basic fibroblast growth factor in rat with Walker-256 transplanted hepatoma: an experimental study. World J Gastroenterol. 2003 Nov 9;9:2445.
33. Lucatelli P, Burrel M, Guiu B, de Rubeis G, Van Delden O. Thomas Helemberg. CIRSE standards of practice on hepatic transarterial chemoembolisation. Cardiovasc Intervent Radiol. 2021;44:1851.
34. Groupe d'Etude et de Traitement du Carcinome Hépatocellulaire. A comparison of lipiodol chemoembolization and conservative treatment for unresectable hepatocellular carcinoma. N Engl J Med. 1995 May 11;332(19):1256–61. https://doi.org/10.1056/NEJM199505113321903.
35. Llovet JM, Bruix J. Systematic review of randomized trials for unresectable hepatocellular carcinoma: chemoembolization improves survival. Hepatology. 2003 Feb;37(2):429–42. https://doi.org/10.1053/jhep.2003.50047.
36. Lewis AL, Gonzalez MV, Lloyd AW, Hall B, Tang Y, Willis SL, et al. DC bead: in vitro characterization of a drug-delivery device for transarterial chemoembolization. J Vasc Interv Radiol. 2006 Feb;17(2):335–42.
37. Lewis AL, Taylor RR, Hall B, Gonzalez MV, Willis SL, Stratford PW. Pharmacokinetic and safety study of doxorubicin-eluting beads in a porcine model of hepatic arterial embolization. J Vasc Interv Radiol. 2006 Aug;17(8):1335–43.
38. Hong K, Khwaja A, Liapi E, Torbenson MS, Georgiades CS, Geschwind JFH. New intra-arterial drug delivery system for the treatment of liver cancer: preclinical assessment in a rabbit model of liver cancer. Clin Cancer Res. 2006 Apr 15;12(8):2563–7.
39. Varela M, Real MI, Burrel M, Forner A, Sala M, Brunet M, et al. Chemoembolization of hepatocellular carcinoma with drug eluting beads: efficacy and doxorubicin pharmacokinetics. J Hepatol. 2007 Mar;46(3):474–81.
40. Poon RTP, Tso WK, Pang RWC, Ng KKC, Woo R, Tai KS, et al. A phase I/II trial of chemoembolization for hepatocellular carcinoma using a novel intra-arterial drug-eluting bead. Clin Gastroenterol Hepatol. 2007;5(9):1100–8.

41. Malagari K, Chatzimichael K, Alexopoulou E, Kelekis A, Hall B, Dourakis S, et al. Transarterial chemoembolization of unresectable hepatocellular carcinoma with drug eluting beads: results of an open-label study of 62 patients. Cardiovasc Intervent Radiol. 2008 Mar;31(2):269–80.
42. de Baere T, Deschamps F, Teriitheau C, Rao P, Conengrapht K, Schlumberger M, et al. Transarterial chemoembolization of liver metastases from well differentiated Gastroenteropancreatic endocrine tumors with doxorubicin-eluting beads: preliminary results. J Vasc Interv Radiol. 2008 Jun;19(6):855–61.
43. Lammer J, Malagari K, Vogl T, Pilleul F, Denys A, Watkinson A, et al. Prospective randomized study of doxorubicin-eluting-bead embolization in the treatment of hepatocellular carcinoma: results of the PRECISION v study. Cardiovasc Intervent Radiol. 2010;33(1):41–52.
44. Irie T. Improved accumulation of lipiodol under balloon-occluded transarterial chemoembolization (B-TACE) for hepatocellular carcinoma: measurement of blood pressure at the embolized artery before and after balloon inflation.
45. Lucatelli P, Ginnani Corradini L, de Rubeis G, Rocco B, Basilico F, Cannavale A, et al. Balloon-occluded Transcatheter arterial chemoembolization (b-TACE) for hepatocellular carcinoma performed with polyethylene-glycol Epirubicin-loaded drug-eluting Embolics: safety and preliminary results. Cardiovasc Intervent Radiol. 2019 Jun 15;42(6):853–62.

2 Transarterial Chemoembolization (TACE): Indications

Laura Crocetti, Paola Scalise, Giulia Lorenzoni, and Elena Bozzi

2.1 Introduction

Transarterial chemoembolization (TACE) represents the standard of care for intermediate-stage hepatocellular carcinoma (HCC) (BCLC stage B) [1]. In this stage, the main aim of TACE is to achieve high overall response (OR) while preserving liver function, which both contribute to prolonging overall survival (OS) and allowing a good quality of life [2, 3]. However, the proper selection of patients is fundamental since the intermediate stage embraces a complex and inhomogeneous population of patients.

Since the positive findings of the first randomized controlled trials (RCTs) and metanalysis that finally demonstrated the positive impact of TACE on survival, it has been the aim of subsequent studies to refine patient selection and technical issues to further improve TACE results as a first-line therapy [4].

In addition, the other main role of TACE is in the setting of liver transplantation (LT): its role in reducing HCC progression as well as a bridge to LT has been well ascertained over the last few years [5].

In modern oncology, the role of locoregional treatments to control tumor progression in liver-dominant disease has gained importance, and transarterial treatments are often taken into consideration in multidisciplinary team discussion for selected patients with cholangiocarcinoma and colorectal, neuroendocrine, and other primary liver metastases [6].

In this chapter, indications for TACE in patients with HCC, as a first-line therapy, and in the pretransplant setting are described. Moreover, indications on how to select patients for non-HCC indication are addressed.

2.2 TACE for Intermediate-Stage HCC

According to the European Association for the Study of the Liver (EASL) guidelines, to the American Association for the Study of Liver Diseases (AASLD) guidelines and in the updated Barcelona Clinic Liver Cancer (BCLC) treatment algorithm, TACE is the current standard of care for intermediate-stage disease (BCLC B) [1, 7, 8] (Table 2.1).

The BCLC stage B includes patients with multinodular HCCs (more than 3 nodules, at least

L. Crocetti (✉)
Division of Interventional Radiology, Azienda Ospedaliero Universitaria Pisana, Pisa, Italy

Department of Surgical, Medical and Molecular Pathology and Critical Care, University of Pisa, Pisa, Italy
e-mail: laura.crocetti@unipi.it

P. Scalise · G. Lorenzoni · E. Bozzi
Division of Interventional Radiology, Azienda Ospedaliero Universitaria Pisana, Pisa, Italy

P. Lucatelli (ed.), *Transarterial Chemoembolization (TACE)*,
https://doi.org/10.1007/978-3-031-36261-3_2

one with diameter larger than 3 cm), without vascular invasion or extrahepatic spread and with well-preserved liver function and performance status. Child-Pugh classification has been recently replaced with the concept of "preserved liver function," a wider concept that includes albumin-bilirubin (ALBI) score, Child Pugh and Mayo End-stage Liver Disease (MELD) [1]. Alpha-fetoprotein (AFP) concentration, regardless of rumor burden, may also impact prognosis and should be therefore included in a more comprehensive patient evaluation [9]. Patient performance status evaluation should also be performed with caution as it may be difficult to differentiate when performance status impairment is related to liver dysfunction, which may or may not be related to tumor burden [1].

Patient population with HCC included in the intermediate stage may have very different tumor burden, which is the reason why the updated BCLC algorithm subdivides this stage in three further subgroups [1].

The first subgroup within BCLC B stage includes patients with well-defined HCC nodules who fit with extended liver transplant criteria according to the criteria of the institution [10]. The second subgroup includes patients without option for LT but who have preserved portal flow and defined tumor burden suggesting the feasibility of selective access to feeding tumor arteries. They are candidates for TACE [1] (Table 2.1).

The third subgroup within BCLC B includes patients with diffuse, infiltrative, extensive HCC liver involvement. They do not benefit from TACE, and systemic therapy should be the recommended option, although there is no strict cut-off when this is the case [11].

Table 2.1 Summary of indications for TACE

HCC stage	Indications
Early stage	• when first treatment options not feasible or failed • in nodules >3 cm and > 5 cm in combination with thermal ablation
Intermediate stage	• multinodular HCC, preserved liver function, PS0, well-defined nodules, selective access possible, preserved portal flow
Bridging to LT	• when time on the waiting list longer than 6 months
Downstaging to LT	• aimed to downstage tumor burden within Milan criteria

PS performance status; *LT* liver transplantation

The Japanese Society of Hepatology (JSH) has recently endorsed criteria to define TACE unsuitability/ineligibility, TACE impossible, and TACE failure [12]. TACE unsuitability/ineligibility generally refers to the following three conditions: (1) likely to develop TACE failure/refractoriness, (2) likely to become Child-Pugh class B liver function after TACE, and (3) unlikely to respond to TACE. Patients likely to develop TACE failure/refractoriness include those who do not meet the up-to-7 criteria in relation to tumor size and number of tumors. Patients prone to reduced liver function include those classified as ALBI grade 2 as well as those who do not meet the up-to-7 criteria (especially bilobar multifocal nodules). Even a single TACE session in a patient with ALBI grade 2 liver function may further reduce liver function, which makes the patient ineligible for systemic therapy with likely shortened OS. Therefore, TACE may be harmful for patients with these conditions. Finally, conditions unlikely to respond to TACE include HCCs with unencapsulated tumors and high incidence of microvascular invasion, such as the simple nodular type with extranodular growth, confluent multinodular type, massive type, infiltrative type, and diffuse type, in addition to poorly differentiated HCCs [12].

Patients are considered TACE impossible upon disappearance/devastation of the feeding artery due to repeated TACE and/or the development of a parasitic feeding artery, which precludes selective catheterization. Patients whose liver function has worsened to Child-Pugh class C after repeated TACE are also considered TACE impossible. Patients with large arterioportal shunts or major vascular invasion such as main portal branches or portal trunk disease are also considered TACE impossible because of the risk of liver failure caused by TACE [12].

The availability of several lines of systemic therapy treatment makes it very important to stop performing TACE in case of nonresponse or progression, in order to not deteriorate liver function and prevent patients to receive systemic therapies. In particular, JSH suggests that TACE should be stopped when two or more consecutive ineffective responses or progression of the disease within the treated tumors (viable lesion >50%) are observed, even after changing the chemotherapeutic agents and/or reanalysis of feeding artery, on response evaluation CT/MRI after 1–3 months following adequately performed selective TACE [12].

Despite a very long history, there is no standard technique regarding all aspects of the procedure including drugs, embolic materials, and microcatheter selection. In the treatment of HCC, doxorubicin is the most used chemotherapeutic agent, although several other drugs are also used, including epirubicin, idarubicin, cisplatin, and mitomycin C. Concerning the embolic material, TACE has classically been performed with an emulsion of Lipiodol and chemotherapeutic drugs followed by Gelfoam (conventional TACE). In the late 2000s, drug-eluting beads (DEB) became available for clinical use and showed a better safety profile with lower systemic drug-related toxicity, although without significant added value on local tumor control over conventional TACE [1, 6, 7].

In this complex scenario, the role of the multidisciplinary team in individualizing treatment strategy is evident. It has been in fact demonstrated that MDT discussion improves patient outcomes and that even when decision is taken in discordance with guidelines but in a patient-tailored manner, the results may ultimately be equal to or even superior to those expected per tumor stage [13, 14].

2.3 TACE for Non-intermediate-Stage HCC

1. In clinical practice, not all patients with early-stage HCC are suitable for curative therapies, such as LT, surgical resection, or ablation due to several clinical factors, such as old age, hepatic dysfunction, tumor location, and comorbidities [7] (Table 2.1).

Despite having early-stage disease, this subset of patients could be good candidates for TACE. This treatment stage-migration strategy is well established and is recommended by international guidelines [1, 7]; several studies have reported a high response rate and good outcomes after TACE in patients with early-stage HCC [6].

A particular subset of patients where TACE is often performed is in combination with thermal ablation in patients with HCC nodules larger than 3 cm. Despite not included in current guidelines, the combination of TACE and radiofrequency ablation is associated with significantly higher overall survival and recurrence-free survival, than radiofrequency monotherapy, without a significant difference in major complications [7] (Table 2.1).

There is not enough evidence in the literature to support the use of TACE for patients in the advanced stage, not even in cases with locally advanced disease such as segmental/sectorial portal vein invasion, where systemic therapies are presently indicated and radioembolization may be discussed as an option at MDT [7].

2.4 TACE for Bridging and Downstaging HCC to LT

Patients with HCC are at high risk of list dropout due to tumor progression while waiting for LT. *Bridging therapy* is intended to prevent dropouts especially if the estimated waiting time is of ≥6 months: in fact, approximately 22% of patients with HCC drop off the waiting list and patients who do not receive any bridging treatments have a 1-year drop-out rate greater than 30% [5]. Several studies have shown that in patients who were bridged to liver transplantation by means of TACE, the drop-out rates were of 3%–9.3%, significantly lower if compared to the ones of the pre-bridging therapy era [5] (Table 2.1).

The term *downstaging* describes treatment used to bring patients whose tumor burden is outside accepted criteria for transplantation to within acceptable criteria. Acceptable criteria are defined as those criteria achieving an expected survival after LT equal to patients who meet transplant criteria without downstaging [5]. According to EASL guidelines, patients are accepted as LT candidates when their HCC, presenting at an intermediate/advanced stage, is successfully down-staged to within the Milan criteria [7]. Patients with HCC initially exceeding Milan criteria and down-staged with TACE can achieve post-transplant survival and HCC recurrence-free probability at 5 years similar to those of patients within Milan criteria [5, 15, 16] (Table 2.1).

Some concerns have been raised about possible impairment of liver function in cirrhotic patients treated with TACE, as well as the increased risk of postoperative hepatic artery complications in patients undergoing TACE before liver transplantation [17, 18]. On the contrary, two recent retrospective studies conducted in transplanted patients who were previously submitted to TACE showed that the incidence of hepatic artery thrombosis was quite similar in those who had or had not received TACE and TACE delivered before liver transplant did not affect complications, patient death, or graft failure after transplantation [19, 20].

When TACE is performed as a neoadjuvant therapy before LT, there is not enough data to establish if it is preferable to use conventional TACE (c-TACE) or DEB-TACE. A recent publication demonstrates that, compared to Lipiodol TACE, DEB-TACE is better tolerated, allowing for reduced hospitalization, and is associated with more durable local tumor control after complete radiological response. These features may be of specific importance if applied to a patient during a possibly long waiting period before LT [21].

2.5 TACE for Liver-Dominant Primary Cholangiocellular and Metastatic Disease

TACE may be considered as a treatment option in selected patients with other primary tumors (intrahepatic cholangiocarcinoma, iCCA) or secondary tumors from colorectal and non-colorectal carcinomas (neuroendocrine, breast, thyroid cancer, melanoma and in oligometastatic disease controlled with systemic treatment), after discussion in a dedicated multidisciplinary team. In these cases, careful pretreatment imaging is needed to confirm the liver only or oligometastatic disease.

Indications for TACE in iCCA include surgically unresectable or inoperable liver tumors with liver-only disease [22].

In the setting of mCRC, patients with liver-limited disease in whom the available chemotherapeutic lines have failed, TACE may be also considered as a treatment option [23].

TACE can also be considered as an alternative therapy to surgical resection of liver metastasis in patients with NET and as an alternative to systemic treatment in those patients with NETs with disease limited to the liver [24].

In all those specific settings, the choice of embolizing material and drug should be part of the multidisciplinary discussion according to liver functional reserve, tumor burden (selective access/lobar approach), molecular profiling of the disease, and previous response to cytotoxic drugs [6].

References

1. Reig M, Forner A, Rimola J, Ferrer-Fàbrega J, Burrel M, Garcia-Criado Á, Kelley RK, Galle PR, Mazzaferro V, Salem R, Sangro B, Singal AG, Vogel A, Fuster J, Ayuso C, Bruix J. BCLC strategy for prognosis prediction and treatment recommendation: the 2022 update. J Hepatol. 2022;76(3):681–93. https://doi.org/10.1016/j.jhep.2021.11.018. Epub 2021 Nov 19
2. Lammer J, Malagari K, Vogl T, Pilleul F, Denys A, Watkinson A, Pitton M, Sergent G, Pfammatter T, Terraz S, Benhamou Y, Avajon Y, Gruenberger T, Pomoni M, Langenberger H, Schuchmann M, Dumortier J, Mueller C, Chevallier P, Lencioni R, Investigators PRECISIONV. Prospective randomized study of doxorubicin-eluting-bead embolization in the treatment of hepatocellular carcinoma: results of the PRECISION V study. Cardiovasc Intervent Radiol. 2010;33(1):41–52. https://doi.org/10.1007/s00270-009-9711-7. Epub 2009 Nov 12
3. Lencioni R, de Baere T, Soulen MC, Rilling WS, Geschwind JF. Lipiodol transarterial chemoembolization for hepatocellular carcinoma: a systematic review of efficacy and safety data. Hepatology. 2016;64(1):106–16. https://doi.org/10.1002/hep.28453. Epub 2016 Mar 7
4. Llovet JM, Bruix J. Systematic review of randomized trials for unresectable hepatocellular carcinoma: chemoembolization improves survival. Hepatology. 2003;37(2):429–42. https://doi.org/10.1053/jhep.2003.50047.

5. Crocetti L, Bozzi E, Scalise P, Bargellini I, Lorenzoni G, Ghinolfi D, Campani D, Balzano E, De Simone P, Cioni R. Locoregional treatments for bridging and Downstaging HCC to liver transplantation. Cancers (Basel). 2021;13(21):5558. https://doi.org/10.3390/cancers13215558.
6. Lucatelli P, Burrel M, Guiu B, de Rubeis G, van Delden O, Helmberger T. CIRSE standards of Practice on hepatic Transarterial chemoembolisation. Cardiovasc Intervent Radiol. 2021;44(12):1851–67. https://doi.org/10.1007/s00270-021-02968-1. Epub 2021 Oct 25
7. Galle PR, Forner A, Llovet JM, Mazzaferro V, Piscaglia F, Raoul J-L, Schirmacher P, Vilgrain V. EASL clinical practice guidelines: management of hepatocellular carcinoma. J Hepatol. 2018;69:182–236. https://doi.org/10.1016/j.jhep.2018.03.019.
8. Heimbach JK, Kulik LM, Finn RS, Sirlin CB, Abecassis MM, Roberts LR, Zhu AX, Murad MH, Marrero JA. AASLD guidelines for the treatment of hepatocellular carcinoma. Hepatology. 2018;67(1):358–80. https://doi.org/10.1002/hep.29086.
9. Singal AG, Hoshida Y, Pinato DJ, Marrero J, Nault JC, Paradis V, Tayob N, Sherman M, Lim YS, Feng Z, Lok AS, Rinaudo JA, Srivastava S, Llovet JM, Villanueva A. International liver cancer association (ILCA) white paper on biomarker development for hepatocellular carcinoma. Gastroenterology. 2021;160(7):2572–84. https://doi.org/10.1053/j.gastro.2021.01.233. Epub 2021 Mar 9
10. Mehta N, Bhangui P, Yao FY, Mazzaferro V, Toso C, Akamatsu N, Durand F, Ijzermans J, Polak W, Zheng S, Roberts JP, Sapisochin G, Hibi T, Kwan NM, Ghobrial M, Soin A. Liver transplantation for hepatocellular carcinoma. Working group report from the ILTS transplant oncology consensus conference. Transplantation. 2020 Jun;104(6):1136–42. https://doi.org/10.1097/TP.0000000000003174.
11. Reig M, Darnell A, Forner A, Rimola J, Ayuso C, Bruix J. Systemic therapy for hepatocellular carcinoma: the issue of treatment stage migration and registration of progression using the BCLC-refined RECIST. Semin Liver Dis. 2014;34(4):444–55. https://doi.org/10.1055/s-0034-1394143. Epub 2014 Nov 4
12. Kudo M, Matsui O, Izumi N, Iijima H, Kadoya M, Imai Y, Okusaka T, Miyayama S, Tsuchiya K, Ueshima K, Hiraoka A, Ikeda M, Ogasawara S, Yamashita T, Minami T, Yamakado K. Liver cancer study group of Japan. JSH consensus-based clinical practice guidelines for the management of hepatocellular carcinoma: 2014 update by the liver cancer study Group of Japan. Liver Cancer. 2014 Oct;3(3–4):458–68. https://doi.org/10.1159/000343875.
13. Sinn DH, Choi GS, Park HC, Kim JM, Kim H, Song KD, Kang TW, Lee MW, Rhim H, Hyun D, Cho SK, Shin SW, Jeong WK, Kim SH, Yu JI, Ha SY, Lee SJ, Lim HY, Kim K, Ahn JH, Kang W, Gwak GY, Paik YH, Choi MS, Lee JH, Koh KC, Joh JW, Lim HK, Paik SW. Multidisciplinary approach is associated with improved survival of hepatocellular carcinoma patients. PLoS One. 2019 Jan 14;14(1):e0210730. https://doi.org/10.1371/journal.pone.0210730.
14. Matsumoto MM, Mouli S, Saxena P, Gabr A, Riaz A, Kulik L, Ganger D, Maddur H, Boike J, Flamm S, Moore C, Kalyan A, Desai K, Thornburg B, Abecassis M, Hickey R, Caicedo J, Grace K, Lewandowski RJ, Salem R. Comparing real world, personalized, multidisciplinary tumor board recommendations with BCLC algorithm: 321-patient analysis. Cardiovasc Intervent Radiol. 2021;44(7):1070–80. https://doi.org/10.1007/s00270-021-02810-8. Epub 2021 Apr 6
15. Mehta N, Frenette C, Tabrizian P, Hoteit M, Guy J, Parikh N, Ghaziani TT, Dhanasekaran R, Dodge JL, Natarajan B, Holzner ML, Frankul L, Chan W, Fobar A, Florman S, Yao FY. Downstaging outcomes for hepatocellular carcinoma: results from the multicenter evaluation of reduction in tumor size before liver transplantation (MERITS-LT) consortium. Gastroenterology. 2021;161(5):1502–12. https://doi.org/10.1053/j.gastro.2021.07.033. Epub 2021 Jul 28
16. Peng CW, Teng W, Lui KW, Hung CF, Jeng WJ, Huang CH, Chen WT, Lin CC, Lin CY, Lin SM, Sheen IS. Complete response at first transarterial chemoembolization predicts favorable outcome in hepatocellular carcinoma. Am J Cancer Res. 2021;11(10):4956–65.
17. Kohla MA, Abu Zeid MI, Al-Warraky M, Taha H, Gish RG. Predictors of hepatic decompensation after TACE for hepatocellular carcinoma. BMJ Open Gastroenterol. 2015;2(1):e000032. https://doi.org/10.1136/bmjgast-2015-000032.
18. Sneiders D, Houwen T, Pengel LHM, Polak WG, Dor FJMF, Hartog H. Systematic review and meta-analysis of Posttransplant hepatic artery and biliary complications in patients treated with Transarterial chemoembolization before liver transplantation. Transplantation. 2018;102(1):88–96. https://doi.org/10.1097/TP.0000000000001936.
19. Wallace D, Cowling TE, Walker K, Suddle A, Gimson A, Rowe I, Callaghan C, Sapisochin G, Mehta N, Heaton N, van der Meulen J. Liver transplantation outcomes after transarterial chemotherapy for hepatocellular carcinoma. Br J Surg. 2020;107(9):1183–91. https://doi.org/10.1002/bjs.11559. Epub 2020 Mar 28
20. Kallini JR, Gabr A, Ali R, Abouchaleh N, Riaz A, Baker T, Kulik L, Caicedo J, Salem R, Lewandowski RJ. Pretransplant intra-arterial liver-directed therapy does not increase the risk of hepatic arterial complications in liver transplantation: a single-center 10-year experience. Cardiovasc Intervent Radiol. 2018;41(2):231–8. https://doi.org/10.1007/s00270-017-1793-z. Epub 2017 Sep 12
21. Bargellini I, Lorenzoni V, Lorenzoni G, Scalise P, Andreozzi G, Bozzi E, Giorgi L, Cervelli R, Scandiffio R, Perrone O, Meccia DV, Boccuzzi A, Daviddi F, Cicorelli A, Lunardi A, Crocetti L, Turchetti G, Cioni R. Duration of response after DEB-TACE compared to lipiodol-TACE in HCC-naïve patients:

a propensity score matching analysis. Eur Radiol. 2021;31(10):7512–22. https://doi.org/10.1007/s00330-021-07905-x. Epub 2021 Apr 19
22. NCCN Clinical Practice Guidelines in Oncology: Hepatobiliary Cancers, Version 1. 2022. Available at: https://www.nccn.org/professionals/physician_gls/pdf/hepatobiliary.pdf. Accessed July 11, 2022.
23. Van Cutsem E, Cervantes A, Adam R, Sobrero A, Van Krieken JH, Aderka D, Aranda Aguilar E, Bardelli A, Benson A, Bodoky G, Ciardiello F, D'Hoore A, Diaz-Rubio E, Douillard JY, Ducreux M, Falcone A, Grothey A, Gruenberger T, Haustermans K, Heinemann V, Hoff P, Köhne CH, Labianca R, Laurent-Puig P, Ma B, Maughan T, Muro K, Normanno N, Österlund P, Oyen WJ, Papamichael D, Pentheroudakis G, Pfeiffer P, Price TJ, Punt C, Ricke J, Roth A, Salazar R, Scheithauer W, Schmoll HJ, Tabernero J, Taïeb J, Tejpar S, Wasan H, Yoshino T, Zaanan A, Arnold D. ESMO consensus guidelines for the management of patients with metastatic colorectal cancer. Ann Oncol. 2016;27(8):1386–422. https://doi.org/10.1093/annonc/mdw235. Epub 2016 Jul 5
24. Pavel M, O'Toole D, Costa F, Capdevila J, Gross D, Kianmanesh R, Krenning E, Knigge U, Salazar R, Pape UF, Öberg K. Vienna consensus conference participants. ENETS consensus Guidelines update for the management of distant metastatic disease of intestinal, pancreatic, bronchial neuroendocrine neoplasms (NEN) and NEN of unknown primary site. Neuroendocrinology. 2016;103(2):172–85. https://doi.org/10.1159/000443167. Epub 2016 Jan 5

3 Access and Material

Stavros Spiliopoulos and Lazaros Reppas

3.1 Access

TACE can be performed via common femoral or radial artery access, although brachial artery or distal transradial access can be also used [1–3]. A transradial access offers the benefit of immediate mobilization/ambulation with minimal bleeding complications and less patient discomfort, and is advised in obese patients with hostile abdomen, those unable to lay flat for a long period of time, or those at high bleeding risk [4, 5]. Both local anesthesia and single-wall arterial access should be performed under ultrasound guidance to minimize pain, access attempts, and complications [6]. For all access types, standard 4–5 Fr x 10 cm sheaths can be used with the relative angiographic catheter diameter. Dedicated access kits with 21 G short-length puncture needles are recommended for transradial access.

Preprocedural study of visceral arteries, vascular anatomy, and tumor supply can minimize procedural time and decrease the risk of nontargeted embolization. Frequent anatomical variations such as right hepatic artery arising from the superior mesenteric artery (SMA) and left hepatic artery arising from the left gastric artery can be easily noted in preprocedural CTA imaging.

3.2 Materials and Technique

Celiac axis and SMA are most frequently catheterized from femoral access with 4- or 5-Fr Cobra, Simmons, or SOS angiographic catheters. For challenging catheterizations, Yashiro tip catheter can also be used. For celiac/SM artery catheterization from transradial access, MPA1, VANSCIE, vertebral, or headhunter angiographic catheters can be used.

5 Fr angiographic catheters demonstrate better steerability than the smaller 4Fr and could be used in challenging celiac or SMA catheterizations. An angled 0.035 hydrophilic guide wire is subsequently and carefully advanced distal into the right hepatic artery in order to advance the angiographic catheter in the common hepatic artery, distal to the origin of the gastroduodenal artery, for adequate support, when possible.

In cases of challenging anatomy with steep angulation and/or in cases in which the hepatic artery originates steeply from the proximal portion of the celiac artery, after catheterization of the celiac trunk, the guidewire can be advanced within the splenic artery. Catheter is exchanged with an angled catheter (VANSCIE, vertebral, or similar) and the common hepatic artery can now

S. Spiliopoulos (✉) · L. Reppas
2nd Department of Radiology, Interventional Radiology Unit, National and Kapodistrian University of Athens, "ATTIKON" University General Hospital, Athens, Greece
e-mail: stavspiliop@med.uoa.gr

P. Lucatelli (ed.), *Transarterial Chemoembolization (TACE)*,
https://doi.org/10.1007/978-3-031-36261-3_3

be catheterized by simultaneously injecting contrast, slowly retrieving and turning the angled catheter just at the origin of the celiac artery. Recently, the "side-hole technique" has also been proposed for challenging angulations, in which a side hole is created at the lesser curvature side of a 5-Fr Cobra catheter and a micro-wire with a microcatheter is subsequently advanced through the side hole [7]. Nevertheless, catheterizing just the ostium of the celiac artery with the mother catheter and using the microcatheter to advance within the feeding vessels always remain a valid option.

Standard or specifically designed for TACE microcatheters (length: 105–150 cm; diameter: 2.0–2.8 Fr; 0.018-inch guidewire compatible) are usually required. Digital subtraction angiography (DSA) of the hepatic arteries should be performed before selective catheterization to depict the target lesion(s) and document free antegrade flow of contrast media, confirming that the catheter is not obstructing the flow. Intraprocedural imaging including 3D angiography with a rotational flat panel detector (cone-beam CT, CBCT) or a combined MDCT angiography system is highly recommended as it has been correlated with less complications, increased technical success, and optimization of clinical outcomes [8–10]. Intraprocedural CBCT/MDCTA imaging enables accurate lesion detection, provides guidance for catheterization, and offers intraprocedural treatment assessment and guidance, as in cases of incomplete tumor embolization, further feeders can be identified and catheterized [11, 12]. For detailed CBCT advantages and clinical applications, refer to Chap. 5.

Superselective catheterization is highly recommended in cases of a single lesion or those with short number of lesions, and feeding arteries should be to minimize the risk of nontargeted embolization, increase the local concentration of chemotherapeutic agent within the tumor, and enhance optimization of clinical outcomes [13]. The materials used in a typical TACE procedure are described in Table 3.1.

Embolic agents should be delivered with the catheter tip beyond the origin of the gastroduodenal artery, the right gastric artery (usually arising from the proper hepatic artery), and the cystic artery (mainly arising from the right hepatic artery) to avoid nontargeted embolization of the bowel, stomach, and gallbladder, respectively. Once the catheter has been positioned at the desired feeding vessel and prior to the delivery of the embolic material, a superselective arteriogram (usually 8–10 ml total contrast volume, 4–5 ml/sec rate, 800 psi) performed via the microcatheter confirms the correct position of the tip as well as the free antegrade flow of contrast media within the tumor but could also depict additional vessels that were not noted during the previous less selective angiograms. It is important that free antegrade flow is demonstrated before infusion, and the physician should be able to visualize that both the macro- and the microcatheter are positioned within adequately sized vessels, as to avoid backflow and guarantee the delivery of the materials within the lesion. Available embolic agents typically used for TACE are presented in Table 3.2. Luer-lock syringes and female/male Luer-lock connections are recommended for safe infusion during DEB-TACE while dedicated Lipiodol-resistant infusion sets can be used for c-TACE.

In the presence of arterio-portal or arterio-venous shunts, selective embolization is suggested. Several embolization materials are

Table 3.1 Recommended materials during a typical TACE procedure

1. Study preprocedural CT (including detailed analysis of the vascular anatomy).
2. Arterial access (US guided under local anesthesia): 4/5 Fr sheath.
3. Celiac axis catheterization and arteriogram (CBCT or MDCTA highly recommended). • 4- or 5-Fr catheter: Cobra Simmons/SOS (femoral access) or VANSCIE/vertebral/headhunter (radial access) • A 0.035 angled hydrophilic guidewire.
4. Superselective catheterization of the feeder(s) and angiogram: • Microcatheter.
5. Embolization/drug delivery: See Table 3.2. • DEB-TACE. • C-TACE (Lipiodol/drug).
6. Hemostasis of vascular access: • 4 Fr: Manual compression • 5–6 Fr: Closure device.

Table 3.2 Embolic agents typically used for TACE

c-TACE: Suspension of Lipiodol and chemotherapy drugs followed by Gelfoam or 100–300 μm embolic particles
DEB-TACE: Drug-eluting microsphere usually 75 μm–300 μm: • DC/LC bead (BTG international, PA, USA). • Hepasphere/Quadrasphere (merit medical, UT, USA). • Tandem/Embozene (Boston Scientific, MA, USA). • LifePearl (Terumo medical, Japan).
Chemotherapy drugs: • HCC: Doxorubicin, epirubicin 75–150 mg per session/doxorubicin, epirubicin, cisplatin, and mitomycin for c-TACE.
Nonionic contrast medium: Usually 5–10 mL/liter of microspheres

available, and the choice should depend on the specific anatomical details and the experience of the physician. N-butyl-2-cyanoacrylate (glue) use has been mainly reported in the literature. The dilution of Lipiodol/N-butyl-2-cyanoacrylate depends on the dimensions and hemodynamic characteristics of the shunt, and generally low-viscosity mixtures are used for high-flow, large shunts, while balloon occlusion techniques have been implemented in order to avoid nontargeted distal embolization [14, 15]. Coils and gelatin sponge (plain or soaked with ethanol) can also be used successfully in selected cases [16].

3.2.1 Novel Anti-Reflux Microcatheters. Pressure-Assisted Embolization

Although typical end-hole microcatheters are currently the standard of TACE therapy, novel-anti-reflux technology has been implemented, aiming in preventing retrograde flow and minimize non-target delivery. This novel class of anti-reflux microcatheters (also called "flow-directed" or "pressure-assisted" microcatheters) uses micro-balloons, valves, or dynamic flow obstruction technology to prevent backflow of the embolic material and enhance intratumoral delivery. Moreover, it has been proposed that pressure-assisted embolization, enabled by anti-reflux microcatheters, results in reduced both extrahepatic and intrahepatic non target embolization, and therefore improves selective intra-tumor delivery, due to a significant reduction in the blood pressure occurring in the downstream antegrade vascular territory and flow redistribution via intra-hepatic collaterals. [17, 18]

Specifically, the Surefire® Infusion System (SIS; TriSalus Life Sciences, USA) is using a patented valve system that partially collapses with forward systolic arterial flow and expands with reversed diastolic flow avoiding reflux during delivery. SIS is introduced through a 5F guiding catheter with an inner diameter of 1.37 mm (0.054 inches) or greater and is available in 3.7 Fr/3.4 Fr proximal distal tip/outer diameter and 120 cm and 150 cm (SIS Radial) usable lengths. Also, two sizes are available (SIS 025M for vessel between -2.0 and 4.0 mm and SIS 025L for vessels between -4.0 and 6.0 mm) [19–21]

The IsoFlow™ dual-balloon anti-reflux microcatheter (Vascular Designs Inc., USA) is equipped with two compliant balloons (can be inflated from 2 to 6 mm), positioned near the distal end of the catheter. Between the two balloons, there is a 10 mm long infusion segment (with multiple side holes). The IsoFlow™ microcatheter has three lumens: one for balloons inflation, one for infusion through the side holes, and a third to accommodate the guidewire (0.014 inch). The IsoFlow™ catheter can be inserted via a 5-Fr guiding catheter, with a 0.056-inch inner diameter. It is available in 150 cm length and a proximal/distal outer diameter of 3.5 F and 2.3 F, respectively, and can deliver embolic materials up to 300 μm [22].

The Occlusafe® Temporary Occlusion Balloon Catheter (Terumo, Japan) is a microcatheter equipped with a single balloon at the distal tip that can be inflated to occlude vessels measuring from 1 mm to 4 mm (balloon inflation minimum volume 0.02 mL and maximum volume 0.10 mL). It is compatible with a 0.014-inch guidewire and available in 110 to 150 cm length. The proximal/distal outer diameter is 2.8 Fr and 2.7 Fr, respectively.

Finally, the SeQure® Reflux Control Microcatheter (Guerbet, Princeton, USA) uses

Table 3.3 Commercially available anti-reflux catheters indicated for TACE

Brand name	Technical characteristics
Surefire® precision infusion system (TriSalus life sciences, USA)	Expandable basket; requires specific angiographic catheters
IsoFlow™ microcatheter (vascular designs Inc., USA)	Dual-balloon technology
Occlusafe® temporary occlusion balloon catheter (Terumo, Japan)	Inflatable balloon
SeQure® reflux control microcatheter (Guerbet, USA)	Dynamic flow obstruction technology

side slits that generate a fluid barrier during infusion impeding reflux of the embolic material. This flow dynamic technology is based on the fact that side slits measure <70 μm size and therefore allow the outflow of contrast media without passage of the embolic microspheres. It is compatible with 0.018- to 0.021-inch guidewires and available in 105 to 150 cm in lengths. The SeQure® microcatheter is available in proximal/distal outer diameters of 2.9/2.4 Fr, 2.9/2.7 Fr, and 3.0/2.8 Fr, delivering embolic microspheres measuring 70–500 μm, 70–500 μm, and 70–700 μm, respectively, but also 0.018-inch micro coils [23].

Commercially available anti-reflux microcatheters indicated for TACE procedures are summarized in Table 3.3.

References

1. Iezzi R, Pompili M, Posa A, et al. Transradial versus transfemoral access for hepatic chemoembolization: intrapatient prospective single-center study. J Vasc Interv Radiol. 2017;28(9):1234–9.
2. Du N, Ma J, Yang M, Zhang Z, Zheng Z, Zhang W, Yan Z. Transradial access chemoembolization for hepatocellular carcinoma patients. J Vis Exp. 2020 Sep;20(163)
3. van Dam L, Geeraedts T, Bijdevaate D, van Doormaal PJ, The A, Moelker A. Distal radial artery access for noncoronary endovascular treatment is a safe and feasible technique. J Vasc Interv Radiol. 2019;30(8):1281–5.
4. Titano JJ, Biederman DM, Zech J, et al. Safety and outcomes of Transradial access in patients with international normalized ratio 1.5 or above. J Vasc Interv Radiol. 2018 Mar;29(3):383–8.
5. Nairoukh Z, Jahangir S, Adjepong D, Malik BH. Distal radial artery access: the future of cardiovascular intervention. Cureus. 2020;12(3):e7201.
6. Spiliopoulos S, Katsanos K, Diamantopoulos A, Karnabatidis D, Siablis D. Does ultrasound-guided lidocaine injection improve local anaesthesia before femoral artery catheterization? Clin Radiol. 2011;66(5):449–55.
7. Meng XX, Liao HQ, Liu HC, et al. Application of side-hole catheter technique for transradial arterial chemoembolization in patients with hepatocellular carcinoma. Abdom Radiol (NY). 2019;44(9):3195–9.
8. Tacher V, Radaelli A, Lin M, Geschwind JF. How I do it: cone-beam CT during transarterial chemoembolization for liver cancer. Radiology. 2015;274(2):320–34.
9. Tacher V, Lin M, Bhagat N, et al. Dual-phase cone-beam computed tomography to see, reach, and treat hepatocellular carcinoma during drug-eluting beads transarterial chemoembolization. J Vis Exp. 2013;82:50795.
10. Loffroy R, Lin M, Yenokyan G, et al. Intraprocedural C-arm dual-phase cone-beam CT: can it be used to predict short-term response to TACE with drug-eluting beads in patients with hepatocellular carcinoma? Radiology. 2013;266(2):636–48.
11. Albrecht MH, Vogl TJ, Wichmann JL, et al. Dynamic 4D-CT angiography for guiding Transarterial chemoembolization: impact on the reduction of contrast material, operator radiation exposure, catheter consumption, and diagnostic confidence. Rofo. 2018 Jun;190(6):513–20.
12. de Baere T, Arai Y, Lencioni R, et al. Treatment of liver tumors with Lipiodol TACE: technical recommendations from experts opinion. Cardiovasc Intervent Radiol. 2016;39(3):334–43.
13. Yamakado K, Miyayama S, Hirota S, et al. Hepatic arterial embolization for unresectable hepatocellular carcinomas: do technical factors affect prognosis? Jpn J Radiol. 2012;30(7):560–6.
14. Duan F, Bai Y, Cui L, Li X, Yan J, Zhu H. Transarterial embolization with N-butyl 2-cyanoacrylate for the treatment of arterioportal shunts in patients with hepatocellular carcinoma. J Cancer Res Ther. 2017;13(4):631–5.
15. Takao H, Shibata E, Ohtomo K. Double-balloon-assisted n-Butyl-2-cyanoacrylate embolization of intrahepatic Arterioportal shunt prior to chemoembolization of hepatocellular carcinoma. Cardiovasc Intervent Radiol. 2016;39(10):1479–83.
16. Zhou WZ, Shi HB, Liu S, et al. Arterioportal shunts in patients with hepatocellular carcinoma treated using ethanol-soaked gelatin sponge: therapeutic effects and prognostic factors. J Vasc Interv Radiol. 2015;26(2):223–30.
17. Morshedi MM, Bauman M, Rose SC, Kikolski SG. Yttrium-90 resin microsphere radioembolization using an antireflux catheter: an alternative to

traditional coil embolization for nontarget protection. Cardiovasc Intervent Radiol. 2015;38(2):381–8.
18. Rose SC, Narsinh KH, Isaacson AJ, Fischman AM, Golzarian J. The beauty and bane of pressure-directed Embolotherapy: hemodynamic principles and preliminary clinical evidence. AJR Am J Roentgenol. 2019;212(3):686–95.
19. Kim AY, Miller A. Evaluation of Surefire's precision direct-to-tumor embolization device to augment therapeutic response to intra-arterial, liver-directed therapies for patients with primary and secondary liver cancers. Expert Rev Med Devices. 2016;13(5):435–43.
20. Rose SC, Narsinh KH, Newton IG. Quantification of blood pressure changes in the vascular compartment when using an anti-reflux catheter during chemoembolization versus Radioembolization: a retrospective case series. J Vasc Interv Radiol. 2017;28(1):103–10.
21. van Roekel C, van den Hoven AF, Bastiaannet R, Bruijnen RCG, Braat AJAT, de Keizer B, Lam MGEH, Smits MLJ. Use of an anti-reflux catheter to improve tumor targeting for holmium-166 radioembolization-a prospective, within-patient randomized study. Eur J Nucl Med Mol Imaging. 2021;48(5):1658–68.
22. Monsky WL, Padia SA, Hardy AH. Dual-balloon infusion microcatheter for selective drug-eluting bead transarterial chemoembolization: initial feasibility study. Diagn Interv Radiol. 2017;23(6):454–60.
23. Lucatelli P, Ginnani Corradini L, et al. Balloon-occluded Transcatheter arterial chemoembolization (b-TACE) for hepatocellular carcinoma performed with polyethylene-glycol Epirubicin-loaded drug-eluting Embolics: safety and preliminary results. Cardiovasc Intervent Radiol. 2019 Jun;42(6):853–62.

4 Preprocedure Workup

Argirò Renato and Gasparrini Fulvio

TACE is an established treatment for patients with intermediate-stage HCC.

The development of new effective diagnostic procedures such as ultrasound, spiral CT, and MRI has led to improved preoperative patient selection and thus improved overall survival.

Correct patient selection and proper preparation of the procedure in each step play a central role in the success of the treatment and the final outcome.

In this chapter, we discuss the current management of patients with HCC undergoing TACE.

Particular emphasis is given to the diagnostic and clinical workup as it should be performed currently. Standard preprocedure workup and periprocedure patient management are also discussed.

4.1 Preprocedure Workup

4.1.1 Outpatient Examination

The outpatient visit is a key step in the pretreatment workup. During the visit, the indications are assessed, the patient informed, and the treatment planned in every step, including additional laboratory analyses and imaging studies.

Much has been written about patient selection and detailed coverage of this area is beyond the scope of this chapter. However, during outpatient visit, certain aspects of patient selection must be recognized, including Child-Pugh classification, extrahepatic involvement, liver tumor burden, serology values, and eventually portal vein patency.

Patients with extrahepatic metastasis may be candidates if hepatic tumor burden is predominant and is the main cause of symptoms.

Caution should be exercised in Child-Pugh class C patients as TACE is poorly tolerated in this group who are prone to hepatic failure. In patients with large hepatic tumor burden, the staging of treatment into two or more sessions might be necessary to avoid hepatic failure. In general, no more than 50% of liver volume should be embolized in a single procedure. Many physicians will not treat tumors that are bigger than 50% of total liver volume. Staged procedures are usually performed at least 2 weeks apart to allow patients to recover. More time may be needed in some patients to return to baseline.

In patients with elevated liver enzymes in addition to increased bilirubin levels, there is a propensity for hepatic failure and TACE may be contraindicated.

If the patient is judged to be suitable for treatment, the outpatient clinic visit is the best moment

A. Renato (✉) · G. Fulvio
UOSD radiologia interventistica–Dipartimento di Biomedicina e prevenzione, Azienda Ospedaliera Universitaria Policlinico Tor Vergata Rome, Rome, Italy

P. Lucatelli (ed.), *Transarterial Chemoembolization (TACE)*,
https://doi.org/10.1007/978-3-031-36261-3_4

Table 4.1 ECOG performance status

Grade	ECOG Performance Status
0	Fully active, able to carry on all pre-disease performance without restriction
1	Restricted in physically strenuous activity but ambulatory and able to carry out work of a light or sedentary nature, e.g., light housework, office work
2	Ambulatory and capable of all self-care but unable to carry out any work activities; up and about more than 50% of waking hours
3	Capable of only limited self-care; confined to bed or chair more than 50% of waking hours
4	Completely disabled; cannot carry on any self-care; totally confined to bed or chair
5	Dead

to inform the patient about the palliative, curative, or bridging nature of the procedure and its complications.

The patient needs to be carefully informed, orally and in writing, about:

- The various available management options, including observation, transarterial treatments or surgery, and their respective advantages and limitations
- The modalities of transarterial treatment and the necessary compliance during the procedure
- The potential complications, for example, accidental damage to the main hepatic artery, a rare risk, which can make transplant challenging and rarely impossible
- The expected decrease in nodule size, usually not associated with complete disappearance
- The possible regrowth over time with need of additional treatment or surgery.
- The need for long-term follow-up

Patients correctly informed of the treatment options, their potential efficacy and side effects, and the therapeutic alternatives will increase the probability that they will be compliant during the procedure and follow-up.

The outpatient visit should include an exhaustive collection of the patient's anamnesis, including concomitant diseases, prior surgeries or liver-directed therapies, allergies, clotting disorders, relevant comorbidities, and pregnancy status.

4.1.1.1 ECOG Performance Status

The Eastern Cooperative Oncology Group (ECOG) Scale of Performance Status [1] (Table 4.1) use standard criteria for measuring how the disease impacts a patient's daily living abilities. It describes a patient's level of functioning in terms of their ability to care for themself, daily activity, and physical ability (walking, working, etc.).

It is also a way for physicians to track changes in a patient's level of functioning as a result of treatment.

The ECOG Performance Status and the Karnofsky Performance Status [2] are two widely used methods to assess the functional status of a patient. Both scales have been in the public domain for many years as ways to classify a patient according to their functional impairment, compare the effectiveness of therapies, and assess the prognosis of a patient.

4.1.1.2 Laboratory Test

A mandatory up-to-date liver function test should be performed within a week of the TACE given the risk of liver ischemia and failure from the procedure.

Lab analysis should include a comprehensive metabolic panel (CMP), platelets, INR, and tumor markers (AFP, CEA).

It is necessary at this point to focus on the hemorrhagic risk of cirrhotic patients and the most correct method of assessing it in order to avoid unnecessary testing.

The risk of periprocedural bleeding in patients with cirrhosis is variable and characteristics unique to cirrhosis, such as presence of advanced Child-Turcotte-Pugh cirrhosis or presence of acute-on-chronic liver failure, contribute greatly to bleeding risk [3]. Furthermore, other factors can enhance or modify procedural bleeding risk in patients with cirrhosis, such as acute kidney injury [4].

There was no direct evidence that conventional laboratory tests, including INR or PLT count, accurately predict bleeding risk in patients with cirrhosis, although in vitro evidence suggests that a PLT count >55,000/mL provides adequate substrate for thrombin generation in patients with cirrhosis [5]. There is no direct clinical evidence supporting PLT count cutoff across various thresholds in predicting bleeding events. Viscoelastic tests (VETs) are an attractive alternative to traditional coagulation testing, as they are dynamic tests that measure clot formation, clot strength, and dissolution over time. VETs have the unique ability to parse out different components of the coagulation system, PLTs, and fibrinolytic system and measure the effective contribution of each to clot formation. In patients with severe thrombocytopenia or coagulopathy undergoing high-risk procedures, decisions about prophylactic blood transfusions should include potential benefits and risks, such as transfusion reactions and alloimmunization. The threshold for severe thrombocytopenia or coagulopathy could not be clearly defined from the literature and remains a matter of clinical judgment. In many cases, clinical care of these patients should be managed in collaboration with an expert hematologist. The utility of PLT counts to predict bleeding in patients with cirrhosis is uncertain, and low PLT counts may reflect progression and severity of the underlying liver disease accompanying portal hypertension, and hypersplenism to a greater extent than bleeding risk at baseline [6]. Despite this, PLTs are commonly transfused in patients with cirrhosis and thrombocytopenia before invasive procedures. This strategy poses some risk to patients, given the short half-life of the transfusions, cost, and the possibility of alloimmunization and other adverse reactions.

4.1.1.3 Imaging

Cross-sectional imaging is mandatory prior to TACE to localize liver tumors, to assess portal vein patency, to look for other comorbid conditions such as bile duct obstruction (which must be decompressed prior to procedure), and to examine arterial anatomy for treatment planning.

The preparation of a patient for TACE includes high-quality triple-phase post-contrast CT to delineate the arterial anatomy and circulation to the tumor or magnetic resonance imaging (MRI) with liver-specific contrast agents.

Radiologists should understand the anatomy of the hepatic vasculature and confirm on conventional angiograms the location of an artery or lesion seen at CT. Embolization of the wrong branch due to lack of a correlated roadmap and lack of familiarity with variants of normal anatomy of liver vasculature can result in inadequate deposition of chemotherapeutic agents in the intended lesion or their unintended distribution. Furthermore, awareness of "mimickers" of segmental branches of the hepatic artery might prevent slow healing and complications such as ulceration of the cystic or gastric wall resulting from arterial embolization in these areas.

Hepatic artery anatomical variations are a common finding. According to publications, normal variant is encountered in 25–80% of individuals. One of the earliest publications regarding liver vascular anatomy belongs to Michels, who divided the variations into 10 variants [7].

According to publications, computed tomography (CT) angiography is the most reliable noninvasive tool to assess arterial anatomy of the liver. Vascular maps could be generated from the processed axial data using multiplanar reformations, maximum intensity projections, curved planar reformations, and volume-rendered technique reconstruction. A willing radiologist could perform the image post-processing to create a 3D reconstruction of the hepatic arteries, portal vein, and hepatic veins.

When the typical pattern of enhancement, consisting of late arterial hyperenhancement followed by washout, is present in nodules larger than 1 cm, HCC can be safely diagnosed without the need for further investigation. However, HCC may show an atypical pattern of enhancement, either as an iso- or hypovascular lesion, or as a hypervascular lesion without washout.

Difficulties in the noninvasive diagnosis of HCC may arise not only because of its atypical enhancement pattern but also because of a variety of morphological growth patterns, different histological subtypes and intralesional complications, such as hemorrhage, necrosis, and cystic degeneration.

In these cases, MRI is the preferred diagnostic modality for the preoperative study of patients with HCC.

MRI has a higher sensitivity for the assessment of the number and location of lesions; however, in the study by Piana et al. [8], MRI had a sensitivity of only 37.1% in the diagnosis of small HCC, and 78.8% in HCC larger than 3 cm, using this typical vascular criterion. A slightly higher sensitivity for the detection of small HCC was reported in the study by Forner et al. [9] (61.7%), since these authors used not only the vascular profile as a diagnostic criterion but also T2-weighted hyperintensity. This compels the integration of more advanced MRI tools, such as hepatospecific contrast agents like gadoxetic acid, and diffusion-weighted imaging (DWI) into the study protocol. The additional value of these methods could be explained by the complexity of hepatocarcinogenesis, which includes changes not only in vascularity but also in architecture, cell density, hepatocyte function, and the number of Kupfer cells. Furthermore, previous studies have shown that HCC with gadoxetic acid uptake is a specific genetic subtype with less aggressive behavior and a better prognosis. In addition, evaluation of the hepatobiliary phase allows assessment of the relationship of the cancer with the major biliary pathways.

Finally, MR has a greater sensitivity in differentiating atypical forms of HCC and portal thrombosis, which are essential elements for correct therapeutic planning [10].

If present, portal vein thrombosis (PVT) does not represent a contraindication if there is adequate collateral flow. The clinical impact of non-tumoral PVT, however, is uncertain and likely reflects the progression of liver disease; whether PVT acts as a precipitant for worsening liver disease is debated. In patients with PVT who undergo TACE, outcomes might be worse, and PVT has been characterized as conveying an increased risk of early mortality [11]. Based on the current literature, there is no direct comparative evidence regarding PVT treatment with anticoagulation and the effects on mortality and/or liver-related morbidity. Furthermore, published studies lack standard bleeding definitions and most did not distinguish portal hypertensive bleeding from other bleeding sources. However, despite the limitations, there is very low certainty evidence that using anticoagulation will promote recanalization and even decrease bleeding.

Importantly, the thrombus itself should not enhance. If enhancement is present, then this strongly suggests that the thrombus is not bland but rather represents tumor thrombus from HCC. The diagnosis can only reliably be made on portal venous phase contrast-enhanced studies. However, the differentiation between bland and tumor thrombus usually requires integrating multiple sequences and taking into account chronicity of the thrombosis.

If the suspicion persists, F-FDG PET/CT including IV iodinated contrast media has demonstrated a promising ability to differentiate between bland thrombus and malignant (tumor thrombus) portal vein thrombosis [12].

Portal involvement is automatically designated as a Barcelona-Clinic Liver Cancer (BCLC) advanced stage "C." TACE is commonly used to treat patients with advanced HCC. Previous studies have demonstrated that TACE had better efficacy than conservative treatment in HCC patients with portal vein tumor thrombosis (PVTT); however, the outcomes of TACE were poor and limited by potential adverse events, high costs, and reduced efficiency [13]. Meanwhile, portal vein wall invasion may lead to thrombi residue and high risk of postoperative recurrence. Tumor thrombus that extends to the main portal vein may lead to extremely poor prognosis due to the following reasons:

- Portal hypertension due to tumor thrombus portal vein obstruction may lead to worse liver function or liver failure, esophageal variceal bleeding, and intractable ascites.
- Extensive intrahepatic metastases due to the tumor cells spread along the portal vein may also contribute to the poor prognosis [14].

The PVTT was graded by using the Shi's classification [15]: tumor thrombus formation was found at microscopic examination, which was defined as Type I0; segmental branches of portal vein or above vein's tumor thrombus, which was defined as Type I; right/left portal vein's tumor thrombus, which was defined as Type II; the main portal vein trunk's tumor thrombus, which was defined as Type III; and the superior mesenteric vein's tumor thrombus, which was defined as Type IV.

4.1.1.4 Echocardiogram

An echocardiogram is performed to assess the left ventricular function and to facilitate both patient selection and assess the impact of cytotoxins on the myocardium, especially if multiple sessions of treatment are being considered.

4.1.1.5 Scores for Initial TACE

The intermediate BCLC group comprises a wide spectrum in terms of liver function and extent of tumor, and this may explain the large differences in survival reported for individual series.

Multiple studies have compared staging systems for their ability to predict the survival of patients treated with TACE, but there is no consensus as to which is best. Scores for initial TACE are extensively explained in Chap. 10.

4.2 Periprocedure Workup

4.2.1 Medications

Before the procedure, patients should be well hydrated with intravenous (IV) fluids such as normal saline 250 cc/h × 4 h and then 150 cc/h × 6 h. This is to reduce the risk of nephrotoxicity from iodinated contrast medium, tumor lysis syndrome, and dehydration due to a lack of fluid intake from postprocedure nausea or vomiting.

Due to the risk of infection and abscess formation, antibiotics for prophylaxis is a routine practice based on the local departmental or hospital rules. Antibiotics, when used, should cover gram-positive, gram-negative, and anaerobic organisms and are recommended for all high-risk patient groups such as diabetics, immunosuppressed, etc. Authors usually use cefoxitin 2 g IV.

If there is a history of biliary surgery, a more aggressive and longer course of antibiotics (10 days) is needed.

Other regimens that cover skin flora and gram-negative enterics are ceftriaxone 1 g, ampicillin/sulbactam (Unasyn) 1.5 g, vancomycin (15 mg/kg) and gentamicin (5 mg/kg) for penicillin allergy and multiple regimens for patients without intact sphincter of Oddi as moxifloxacin 400 mg day x 20 days beginning regimen 3 days before procedure.Other medications useful in managing post-embolization syndrome and reducing pain and nausea are Zofran 10 mg IV push (IVP), Reglan 1 mg IVP, or Decadron 10 mg IV.

4.2.2 Patient Management and Monitoring

Standard monitoring during TACE should include pulse oximetry, ECG, and noninvasive blood pressure. Processed EEG devices may be useful to avoid excessive sedation but are not mandatory. A venous access is mandatory preferably at least 20 G, to allow for rapid IV infusion if needed, whereas in cases of patients with significant coronary disease or other cardiac conditions such as congestive heart failure, the operator may want to consider the placement of an arterial line.

Table 4.2 summarizes the main equipment that the authors recommend should be present in an environment where TACE procedures are performed.

Patient comfort is central to safety during TACE. If patients are comfortable, they are more likely to remain still and follow breathing instructions during vessel navigation, decreasing risk of complications. When patients are sedated, a fine line exists between pain control and ability to follow instructions during embolization. Optimally, patients should be sedated deep enough to be comfortable and experience a light sleep but light enough to follow breathing instructions for accurate catheterization throughout the procedure.

Table 4.2 Minimum mandatory anesthesia equipment for TACE procedure

Airway management equipment:
Oxygen source with flowmeter (preferably wall-mount and with back-up system)
Nasal cannula (preferable with capnography capability) and nonrebreather mask
Bag valve mask and oropharyngeal airway
Second-generation supraglottic airway device (several measures) and equipment for emergent endotracheal intubation
Endotracheal tubes (several measures)
Laryngoscope blades and stylets
Monitoring system:
Pulse oximetry, ECG, noninvasive blood pressure
Temperature probe
Medications:
Sedatives (midazolam, propofol, dexmedetomidine, ketamine)
Opioids (fentanyl, remifentanil, morphine)
Neuromuscular blocking agent (succinylcholine, rocuronium, cisatracurium)
Antagonists (naloxone, flumazenil, neostigmine, sugammadex)
Basic drug for life support (atropine, ephedrine, epinephrine)
Other equipment:
Suction source and catheters
Automated infusion pump defibrillator with paddles

Hence, mild conscious sedation (e.g., midazolam 1–3 mg intravenously) may be useful to keep the patient relaxed during the procedure and allow the operator to communicate during the procedure.

Many authors prefer to perform the procedure under general anesthesia. It avoids patients' movements during the procedure and even achieves a controlled breath-hold that enhances the targeting of the tumor and decreases the risk of dissection or unintended out-target embolization.

In both cases, placement of a bladder Foley catheter to gravity is necessary.

It is essential to position patients appropriately for safety and to spend time assessing patient comfort to ensure immobilization during the procedure. A comfortable, well-positioned patient will remain still during the procedure ensuring correct control of the embolization.

The patient should be placed in a supine position with the apex of the patient's head at the top of the operating bed.

Finally, sufficient space in the room should always be allocated to the anesthetist and all anesthesia equipment to facilitate emergency maneuvers.

Generally, after the procedure, all patients go to the unit after 2 h of supervision.

4.2.3 Expert Nurse Team

Patient comfort is central to safety during TACE and nurses possess the ability to create a safe and comfortable environment for these patients. Thus, nurses have a role in the pre-, intra-, and postprocedural care of patients undergoing TACE.

Prior to the procedure, nurses should check all equipment for proper working order.

Heart rate, respiratory rate, and oxygen saturation should be monitored continuously and blood pressure recorded at least every 5 min throughout the procedure.

Nurses should anticipate giving IV fluids and conscious sedation (usually with midazolam) as ordered. Optimally, patients should be sedated to relieve anxiety after the initial vital signs have been recorded and the sterile area is being prepped but prior to the local skin injection of lidocaine and vessel navigation.

Nurses play a central part to improve outcomes by being aware of their role in care of patients receiving TACE.

References

1. Oken MM, Creech RH, Davis TE. Toxicology and response criteria of the Eastern Cooperative Oncology Group. Am J Clin Oncol Cancer Clin Trials. 1982;5(6):649–55.
2. Karnofsky D, Burchenal J. The clinical evaluation of chemotherapeutic agents in cancer. In: Evaluation of chemotherapeutic agents. 1949.
3. Fisher C, Patel VC, Stoy SH, Singanayagam A, Adelmeijer J, Wendon J, et al. Balanced haemostasis with both hypo- and hyper-coagulable features in critically ill patients with acute-on-chronic-liver failure. J Crit Care. 2018;43:54–60.
4. Hung A, Garcia-Tsao G. Acute kidney injury, but not sepsis, is associated with higher procedure-related

bleeding in patients with decompensated cirrhosis. Liver Int. 2018;38(8):1437–41.
5. Tripodi A, Primignani M, Chantarangkul V, Clerici M, Dell'Era A, Fabris F, et al. Thrombin generation in patients with cirrhosis: the role of platelets. Hepatology. 2006;44(2):440–5.
6. Basili S, Raparelli V, Napoleone L, Talerico G, Corazza GR, Perticone F, et al. Platelet count does not predict bleeding in cirrhotic patients: results from the PRO-LIVER Study. Am J Gastroenterol. 2018;113(3):368–75.
7. Michels NA. Newer anatomy of the liver and its variant blood supply and collateral circulation. Am J Surg. 1966;112(3):337–47.
8. Piana G, Trinquart L, Meskine N, Barrau V, Van BB, Vilgrain V. New MR imaging criteria with a diffusion-weighted sequence for the diagnosis of hepatocellular carcinoma in chronic liver diseases. J Hepatol. 2011;55(1):126–32.
9. Forner A, Vilana R, Ayuso C, Bianchi L, Solé M, Ayuso JR, et al. Diagnosis of hepatic nodules 20 mm or smaller in cirrhosis: prospective validation of the noninvasive diagnostic criteria for hepatocellular carcinoma. Hepatology. 2008;47(1):97–104.
10. Kovac JD, Milovanovic T, Dugalic V, Dumic I. Pearls and pitfalls in magnetic resonance imaging of hepatocellular carcinoma. World J Gastroenterol. 2020;26(17):2012–29.
11. W.M. J, Z. A. TACE in HCC with Portal vein thrombosis. Hepatol Int. 2019;
12. Wu B, Zhang Y, Tan H, Shi H. Value of 18 F-FDG PET/CT in the diagnosis of portal vein tumor thrombus in patients with hepatocellular carcinoma. Abdom Radiol. 2019;44(7):2430–5.
13. Takayasu K, Arii S, Ikai I, Omata M, Okita K, Ichida T, et al. Prospective cohort study of Transarterial chemoembolization for unresectable hepatocellular carcinoma in 8510 patients. Gastroenterology. 2006;131(2):461–9.
14. Peng ZW, Guo RP, Zhang YJ, Lin XJ, Chen MS, Lau WY. Hepatic resection versus transcatheter arterial chemoembolization for the treatment of hepatocellular carcinoma with portal vein tumor thrombus. Cancer. 2012;118(19):4725–36.
15. Shi J, Lai ECH, Li N, Guo WX, Xue J, Lau WY, et al. Surgical treatment of hepatocellular carcinoma with portal vein tumor thrombus. Ann Surg Oncol. 2010;17(8):2073–80.

5 CBCT and Software

Gianluca De Rubeis, Gennaro Castiello, Maria Silvia Giuliani, Pascale Roberte Riu, Sebastiano Fabiano, and Roberto Cianni

5.1 CBCT

5.1.1 Introduction

Cone-beam computed tomography (CBCT) was developed in the early 80 s by the Biodynamics Research Unit at the Mayo Clinic for developing "high temporal resolution and synchronous volume scanning" [1]. Over the past 40 years, CBCT has evolved in two directions: aided interventional radiology (IR) procedures and in oral/maxillofacial radiology [2]. These two streams were developed for two different reasons, in particular, in the set of interventional radiology procedures, for the possibility to supply unique planning and prognostic information and, concerning oral/maxillofacial radiology, for high-quality images, compact size, low cost, and low-ionizing radiation [2].

Technically, images are produced by a rotation of the x-ray source/detector over a fixed point, namely, the region of interest, with the same principle of standard computed tomography (CT) [2, 3]. The principal difference between CBCT and CT is the geometry of the ionized radiation beam [3]. In particular, the configuration of the x-ray source of CBCT is a pyramid (conic) shape; conversely, the one of CT is fan-beam/spiral [3]. The general advantages of CBCT over CT are increased sharpness, reduced image distortion, and increased tube efficiency. In the field of IR, to these advantages is added the possibility of performing cross-sectional imaging directly in the angiographic suite. The main disadvantage is a reduction of contrast to noise ratio due to the presence of large amount of scattered radiation [3]. Four different vendors apply cone-beam technology to C-arm directly in angiographic suite: DynaCT (Siemens, Forchheim, Germany), XperCT (Phillips, Eindhoven, The Netherlands), LCI Cone-Beam CT (Canon Medical, Ōtawara, Japan), and Innova CT (GE Medical Systems, Waukesha, Wisconsin, USA) [4]. Over the years, several applications were developed for CBCT for aided interventional radiologists during procedures. In this section, we discuss the application of this relatively new technology into the field of transarterial chemoembolization (TACE).

5.1.2 Technique Principles

The source of radiation is a flat panel made by amorphous silicon thin-film transistor [5]. In the case of CBCT in the field of IR and, more specifically, for the purpose of the chapter of liver embolization, the complex source/detector of radiation is equipped on an angiographic suite

G. De Rubeis · G. Castiello · M. S. Giuliani
P. R. Riu · S. Fabiano · R. Cianni (✉)
Dipartimento delle Diagnostiche, Azienda Ospedaliera San Camillo Forlanini Hospital, Rome, Italy
e-mail: RCianni@scamilloforlanini.rm.it

P. Lucatelli (ed.), *Transarterial Chemoembolization (TACE)*,
https://doi.org/10.1007/978-3-031-36261-3_5

that is able to rotate around the patients. During the rotation, the flat panel performs a great amount of projection around the region of interest (e.g., the liver) with a rotation of 180° plus the angle of the flat panel reaching at least 200 degrees [6–8]. The acquisition is performed in a pulsating way every 0.39–0.52° with a pitch of 200–800 micron at 15–60 frames per second [7, 9]. The multiple 2D images acquired are directly sent and processed to a 3D reconstruction system. After that, using Parker weighting and correction methods, the 3D images are reconstructed [6, 9]. The flat panel rotates with phases of acceleration and deceleration [9]. Generally, tube voltage ranges from 90 kV to 120 kV with a copper filtration at 30–60 ms as frames rate and pulse width of 5.0 ms [4, 9]. The dimension of the detector is 30 × 40 cm with a spatial resolution of 150 μm² [10]. The resulting spatial resolution achievable is an isotropic voxel of 0.5 mm³ [9], which is comparable with clinical state-of-the-art computed tomography (0.5–0.625 mm) [11, 12]. This spatial resolution is sufficient for 3D isotropic images with the possibility to manipulate the acquired volume in all geometrical planes. Images are reconstructed with filtered back projections [9].

5.1.3 Patient Preparation

In the field of liver embolization assisted by CBCT, the flat panel should rotate over the liver. However, the liver is not in the isocenter of the human body. For this reason, the patient should be laterally (left) positioned to ensure that the isocenter of the CBCT acquisition is the liver [9]. All radiopaque objects should be carefully removed such as ECG leads and cables, pressure cuffs, etc. [9].

5.1.4 Radiation Dose Principle and Concern

The radiation parameter taken into account for dosimetry in CBCT is the dose area product (DAP) [13]. DAP is defined as the amount of radiation dose administered to the skin surface in the region of interest, and it is measured in Gy × cm² [13]. On average, the radiation dose per frame was 0.36 μGy [4]. Anyhow, Suzuki et al. [14], using Monte Carlo simulation, demonstrated that the coefficient to calculate the effective dose is vendor based. A state-of-the-art CBCT permits an abdomen scan using 3–10 mSv [6], which is comparable with a CT scan of the same region. Interestingly, for multiple CBCT acquisitions (e.g., dual-phase CBCT) with the C-arm rotating in both clockwise and counterclockwise directions, the radiation dose cannot be "simply" double due to different geometry and angle of incidence of the x-ray beam [15]. However, under the light of the general principle on radiation dose administration (as low as reasonably achievable [ALARA] [16]), the use of "additional" CBCT for performing interventional radiology has been given some concerns. In fact, although CBCT is able to provide planning and prognostic additional information compared with traditional digital subtraction angiography (DSA)-assisted procedures, the dose administered is significantly higher (increase of about 34%) [6, 17]. However, the augment dose depends on the expertise of the operator ranging from +7.5% (expert) to +75% (novice) [17]. Thus, the ALARA-balance relies upon the value of added info given by CBCT and the "supplementary" radiation dose administered.

5.1.5 Application in Transarterial Chemoembolization

Several different technical variations of CBCT acquisition may be performed depending on angiographic catheter position, time of contrast media injection, and delayed time of the acquisition (see Table 5.1 for details).

5.1.5.1 CBCT during Hepatic Artery Injection

When performing a proper liver arterial phase during CBCT, the diagnostic angiographic catheter (4/5 Fr) should be positioned into the hepatic artery (proper or common) or in the

Table 5.1 Protocols for different applications of CBCT

	Amount (ml)/ rate of contrast (ml/s)	Delay of scan (s)	Vascular detection	Nodules detection	Sensitivity	Specificity	Prognostic value
Basal CBCT	No	End procedure	No	No	No	No	Yes
Arterial CBCT	12–64/4	2–6	Yes	Yes	90%	No	Yes
Dual-phase CBCT	45/4	8 (arterial)/35 (portal)	Yes	Yes	98%	79%	Yes
Portography CBCT	40/3	20	No	Yes	93%	No	No
Perfusion CBCT	α	α	Yes	Yes	α	α	Yes°

CBCT cone-beam computed tomography; *α* since the acquisition is the same as dual-phase CBCT, the results are the same; ° diagnostic accuracy for residual is 79.66% (95% CI, 69.39–89.93%)

celiac trunk with an injection of 12–64 ml of contrast media with a delayed in acquisition of 2–6 seconds with a flow rate of 4/5 ml/s [6, 18]. CBCT in arterial phase is generally performed to depict tumor's vascularization and to detect target nodules [19]. More specifically from the side of tumor's vascularization analysis, CBCT in the arterial phase allows subsegmental chemoembolization without further angiographic studies in 84.9% of patients [20].

In addition, CBCT can identify adjunctive feeder vessels over DSA alone [21], with a pooled sensitivity for feeder's detection of 93% (95% CI, 91–95%) and a pooled specificity of 89% (95% CI, 84–93%) [22].

About the tumor detection rate, the pooled sensitivity is 90% (95% CI, 82–95%), which decreases to 77% for small nodules (<1 cm) [22]. However, these results derive from a meta-analysis with a high degree of heterogeneity (p = 0.001 for homogeneity Q test; I^2 = 92%) [22]. Thus, the CBCT outperforms DSA for tumor detection with dimension >3 cm and the high-contrast resolution images and 3D reconstruction are helpful also for smaller nodules [22].

5.1.5.2 Dual-Phase CBCT

For dual-phase CBCT (DP-CBCT), the angiographic catheter should be posed into the hepatic artery or celiac trunk with an injection of 18–60 ml of a mix of 1/3 of contrast media and saline solution (for avoiding streak artifact) at 4 ml/s flow rate [6, 23]. The injection should last at least 15 seconds for covering both vascular and tumor enhanced [24].

The first CBCT acquisition should start at 8 seconds after the injection, followed by a second acquisition at 35 seconds. This timing of acquisitions permits three different evaluations: in the arterial phase, liver vasculature mapping and tumor enhancement, whereas liver parenchymal ("portal" phase) enhancement is evaluated in the portal phase one [24]. The major advantage of DP-CBCT over single arterial-phase CBCT is the possibility to characterize the nature of the hypervascular focal lesion [24]. The arterial phase is able to detect the lesion (sensitivity), and its behavior on portal phase can classify the focal lesion (specificity) by applying the LI-RADS criteria [19, 24, 25]. Using DP-CBCT, the sensitivity and specificity for hypervascular focality in the liver are 98% and 79%, respectively. In addition, the performance is sufficiently good also for the lesion <1 cm, which is a known dimension limit of multidetector computed tomography and magnetic resonance imaging with potential implication for treatment strategy [24, 26].

DP-CBCT performed after TACE can be useful to predict the HCC response at 1-month MRI follow-up with an excellent degree of correlation (R = 0.89 for arterial phase and second R = 0.82 for portal phase) [15]. Moreover, considering degradable starch microsphere procedures, which consist in repeated procedures over fixed time, DP-CBCT may predict intraprocedural 1-month outcome by comparing the relative enhancement in two different acquisitions [27].

5.1.5.3 CBCT without Contrast Media

CBCT without contrast media injection is generally performed after liver embolization procedure for assessing post-procedural outcome. The capability to observe the embolizing material after TACE depends on its nature (degradable starch microsphere vs Lipidiol vs drug-eluting microsphere). In fact, only Lipidiol (Guerbet, France) and radiopaque beads (LC Bead LUMI; Biocompatibles UK, Farnham, England) are intrinsically hyperdense and can be visible on basal CBCT. On the contrary, the possibility to observe the results of the embolization performed with degradable starch microspheres and radiotransparent beads relies upon their binding with contrast media [23, 28]. The evaluation of Lipiodol deposit on basal CBCT is able to predict 1-month outcome and incomplete area of embolization [29, 30]. The accuracy for detecting viable nodules for CBCT after conventional TACE is 0.816 (vs unenhanced CT of 0.841; $p = 0.449$), with a sensitivity of 80.5%, specificity of 74.2%, and positive (47.5%) and negative (92.9%) [22]. Suk et al. [31] demonstrated that marginal contrast saturation, evaluated in CBCT, is correlated with tumor response at 1 month in hepatocellular carcinoma (HCC). In addition, basal CBCT can identify the filling defects of tumor's contrast material retention, allowing immediate treatment adjustment [28].

5.1.5.4 CBCT during Portography

The angiographic catheter should be positioned into the superior mesenteric artery with an injection of 40 ml of contrast media with dilution at 3 ml/s after the administration of 2.5 μg of prostaglandin E [32]. The CBCT starts 20 s after the injection of contrast media with 621 images acquired in 20 seconds with a rotation of 207° [32]. The physiological principle is based on the liver portal return consisting into the portal vein liver supply following the injection into the mesenteric artery. The HCC is relatively hypoenhanced compared with liver parenchyma [6]. The clue of CBCT portography is the sole detection of liver nodules with a sensitivity range from 93.9% to 100% compared with MDCT [4, 24].

5.1.5.5 CBCT Perfusion

CBCT perfusion is an "evolution" of DP-CBCT by post-processing subtracted mask images and DP-CBCT with a color-coded vendor-specific algorithm based on perfusion degree [33]. Several perfusion parameters can be derived, such as parenchymal blood volume (PBV) [34], PBV mean, and PBV max [33]. The theoretical advantage is that perfusion imaging may overcome the limitation of DP-CBCT, concerning the evaluation of post-procedural outcome, including contrast media heterogeneity or Lipidiol deposition (in case of conventional TACE) [33]. Syha et al. [34] demonstrated that PBV and PBV map can predict tumor response for all treated lesions. Moreover, PBV max and perfusion map independently predict TACE outcome with a diagnostic accuracy of 79.66% (95% CI, 69.39–89.93%) [35]. In addition, the area under the curve, for tumor residual detection, of PBV max is 0.7523, with 80.8% sensitivity and 60.6% specificity [35]. However, this application of CBCT is still an initial research with little but promising body of evidence.

5.1.5.6 Potential Clinical Implication of CBCT

All systems for staging take into account two aspects of liver disease: the number of nodules and the underlying hepatic disease [26, 36, 37]. Based on this evidence, the possibility to detect more HCC may impact clinical decisions [22]. For example, Lucatelli et al. [24] demonstrated that 3/54 (5.5%) of occult HCC >1 cm were depicted in the other hepatic lobe with respect to the target lesion, which may dramatically change the management of the patients (e.g., hepatic lobectomy). Furthermore, the presence of occult nodules have a potential impact also in the transplantation setting. In fact, all transplantation criteria [38] are based on the numbers of HCC. Therefore, the possibility to detect occult HCC may change the approach to the management of the patient and to the inclusion in the transplantation list. Anyhow, at the moment, no studies compared the treatment outcome or transplantation survival in patients with and without occult HCC.

5.2 Software Guidance

5.2.1 Introduction

In recent years, several vendors started producing software for tumor's feeder detection [39–41], such as EmboGuide (Philips Healthcare, Best, The Netherlands), syngo Embolization Guidance (Siemens, Forchheim, Germany), and Flight Plan for Liver (GE Healthcare, Waukesha, WI, USA).

5.2.2 Applications

According to a meta-analysis [42], the application of the embolization-aided software mostly evaluated hepatocellular carcinoma (98.6%) while the remaining on neuroendocrine and metastasis.

In general, the reported sensitivity for feeder detection ranges from 86% (127/147) to 97.1% (66/68) [42]. More specifically, software were compared both with DSA and CBCT with a sensitivity for feeder vessels of 60.5% (95% CI, 38.4–82.5%) and 75.7% (95% CI, 64.0–87.3%), respectively. To the authors' knowledge, there is no direct comparison between embolization-aided softwares. However, single studies were conducted vs DSA and CBCT. In particular, EmboGuide has a sensitivity of 95.6% vs DSA (56.5%) and 86% vs CBCT (86%) [43, 44], and Flight Plan for Liver has a sensitivity of 92.7% vs DSA (85.3%) and 87.7–93% vs CBCT (71.8–81%) [40].

Only two studies compare intraprocedural impact of embolization-aided software. However, the results of these studies are not homogeneous. The study by Cornelis et al. demonstrated reduction of the dose-area product (149.75 Gy*cm2 vs 227.8 Gy*cm2; $p = 0.05$) between "traditional" TACE and embolization-aided software without reduction of the number of DSA and fluoroscopy time [39]. On the contrary, Yao et al. [45] demonstrated more superselective embolization (60% vs 49%), less number of DSA (2.6 ± 0.8 vs 3.4 ± 0.7; $P < 0.001$), shorter fluoroscopy time (4.1 ± 2.6 vs 7.1 ± 4.2 minutes; $P < 0.001$), and increased DAP (134 [95% CI, 92–181] Gy·cm^2 vs 97 [95% CI, 75–140] Gy·cm^2; $P = 0.048$).

In a recent communication, Soliman et al. [46] suggested a new improvement for embolization-aided software. In fact, although the current software helps to map the vasculature of the tumor, a simulation of the distribution of chemoembolization material during a real injection is still a matter of research. In other words, since the clue of TACE is not to reach the tumor but to inject the mixture of chemo drugs and the embolizing material directly into the lesion without other nontarget embolization, this new embolization-aided software allows to simulate a virtual injection and its effect. Liver ASSIST V.I. (GE Healthcare, Chicago, Illinois) [46] allows to simulate the injection from the tip of the catheter to assess the correct final position, providing a more detailed tumor-vasculature map system. Moreover, Ortiz et al. [47] demonstrated an adjunctive use of Liver ASSIST V.I. by superimposing the map with the follow-up cross-sectional imaging to discover the feeder vessel of the residual tumor.

5.2.2.1 Conclusion

CBCT and modern software are able to help interventional radiologists during TACE procedures. Although TACE could be performed without the assistance of CBCT and embolization-aided software, both these tools may add significant benefit to the procedure. In particular, CBCT, independent from contrast injection and time of acquisition, amplified the success of the procedure by including feeder and tumor detection and prognostic factors. Moreover, embolization-aided software helps to determine tumor vasculature map.

In the future, the TACE 2.0 procedure will encompass pre-embolization CBCT for tumor and feeder detection, embolization-aided software for vasculature map, and post-procedural CBCT for prognostic factor.

References

1. Robb RA. The dynamic spatial Reconstructor: an X-ray video-fluoroscopic CT scanner for dynamic volume imaging of moving organs. IEEE Trans Med Imaging. 1982;1(1):22–33.
2. Venkatesh E, Elluru SV. Cone beam computed tomography: basics and applications in dentistry. J Istanb Univ Fac Dent. 2017;51(3 Suppl 1):S102–21.
3. Scarfe WC, Farman AG. What is cone-beam CT and how does it work? Dent Clin N Am. 2008;52(4):707–30. v
4. Tognolini A, et al. C-arm computed tomography for hepatic interventions: a practical guide. J Vasc Interv Radiol. 2010;21(12):1817–23.
5. Yorkston J, Rowlands J. Flat panel detectors for digital radiography. 2000.
6. Tacher V, et al. How I do it: cone-beam CT during Transarterial chemoembolization for liver cancer. Radiology. 2015;274(2):320–34.
7. Lucatelli P, et al. Single injection dual phase CBCT technique ameliorates results of trans-arterial chemoembolization for hepatocellular cancer. Transl Gastroenterol Hepatol. 2017;2:83.
8. Shaw CC. Cone beam computed tomography. Taylor & Francis; 2014.
9. Floridi C, et al. C-arm cone-beam computed tomography in interventional oncology: technical aspects and clinical applications. Radiol Med. 2014;119(7):521–32.
10. Grass M, et al. Three-dimensional reconstruction of high contrast objects using C-arm image intensifier projection data. Comput Med Imaging Graph. 1999;23(6):311–21.
11. Lin E, Alessio A. What are the basic concepts of temporal, contrast, and spatial resolution in cardiac CT? J Cardiovasc Comput Tomogr. 2009;3(6):403–8.
12. Wang J, Fleischmann D. Improving spatial resolution at CT: development, benefits, and pitfalls. Radiology. 2018;289(1):261–2.
13. Miller DL, et al. Quality improvement guidelines for recording patient radiation dose in the medical record for fluoroscopically guided procedures. J Vasc Interv Radiol. 2012;23(1):11–8.
14. Suzuki S, et al. Evaluation of effective dose during abdominal three-dimensional imaging for three flat-panel-detector angiography systems. Cardiovasc Intervent Radiol. 2011;34(2):376–82.
15. Loffroy R, et al. Intraprocedural C-arm dual-phase cone-beam CT: can it be used to predict short-term response to TACE with drug-eluting beads in patients with hepatocellular carcinoma? Radiology. 2013;266(2):636–48.
16. The 2007 Recommendations of the International Commission on Radiological Protection. ICRP publication 103. Ann ICRP, 2007. 37(2–4): p. 1–332.
17. Kothary N, et al. Imaging guidance with C-arm CT: prospective evaluation of its impact on patient radiation exposure during transhepatic arterial chemoembolization. J Vasc Interv Radiol. 2011;22(11):1535–43.
18. Lee IJ, et al. Cone-beam CT hepatic arteriography in chemoembolization for hepatocellular carcinoma: angiographic image quality and its determining factors. J Vasc Interv Radiol. 2014;25(9):1369–79. quiz 1379-e1
19. Mitchell DG, et al. LI-RADS (liver imaging reporting and data system): summary, discussion, and consensus of the LI-RADS Management working group and future directions. Hepatology. 2015;61(3):1056–65.
20. Lee IJ, et al. Cone-beam computed tomography (CBCT) hepatic arteriography in chemoembolization for hepatocellular carcinoma: performance depicting tumors and tumor feeders. Cardiovasc Intervent Radiol. 2015;38(5):1218–30.
21. Ushijima Y, et al. Detecting hepatic nodules and identifying feeding arteries of hepatocellular carcinoma: efficacy of cone-beam computed tomography in transcatheter arterial chemoembolization. Hepatoma Res. 2016;2:231–6.
22. Pung L, et al. The role of cone-beam CT in Transcatheter arterial chemoembolization for hepatocellular carcinoma: a systematic review and meta-analysis. J Vasc Interv Radiol. 2017;28(3):334–41.
23. Mikhail AS, et al. Mapping drug dose distribution on CT images following Transarterial chemoembolization with radiopaque drug-eluting beads in a rabbit tumor model. Radiology. 2018;289(2):396–404.
24. Lucatelli P, et al. Intra-procedural dual phase cone beam computed tomography has a better diagnostic accuracy over pre-procedural MRI and MDCT in detection and characterization of HCC in cirrhotic patients undergoing TACE procedure. Eur J Radiol. 2020;124:108806.
25. Abdel Razek AAK, et al. Liver imaging reporting and data system version 2018: what radiologists need to know. J Comput Assist Tomogr. 2020;44(2):168–77.
26. EASL Clinical Practice Guidelines. Management of hepatocellular carcinoma. J Hepatol. 2018;69(1):182–236.
27. Lucatelli P, et al. Sequential dual-phase cone-beam CT is able to intra-procedurally predict the one-month treatment outcome of multi-focal HCC, in course of degradable starch microsphere TACE. Radiol Med. 2019;124(12):1212–9.
28. Lucatelli P, et al. Are radiopaque beads a real advantage? Radiology. 2019;290(3):852.
29. Orlacchio A, et al. Role of cone-beam CT in the intra-procedural evaluation of chemoembolization of hepatocellular carcinoma. J Oncol. 2021;2021:8856998.
30. Iwazawa J, et al. C-arm CT for assessing initial failure of iodized oil accumulation in chemoembolization of hepatocellular carcinoma. Am J Roentgenol. 2011;197(2):W337–42.

31. Suk Oh J, et al. Transarterial chemoembolization with drug-eluting beads in hepatocellular carcinoma: usefulness of contrast saturation features on cone-beam computed tomography imaging for predicting short-term tumor response. J Vasc Interv Radiol. 2013;24(4):483–9.
32. Miyayama S, et al. Detection of hepatocellular carcinoma by CT during arterial portography using a cone-beam CT technology: comparison with conventional CTAP. Abdom Imaging. 2009;34(4):502–6.
33. Kim KA, et al. The efficacy of cone-beam CT-based liver perfusion mapping to predict initial response of hepatocellular carcinoma to transarterial chemoembolization. J Vasc Interv Radiol. 2019;30(3):358–69.
34. Syha R, et al. Parenchymal blood volume assessed by C-arm-based computed tomography in immediate posttreatment evaluation of drug-eluting bead Transarterial chemoembolization in hepatocellular carcinoma. Investig Radiol. 2016;51(2):121–6.
35. Choi SY, et al. Usefulness of cone-beam ct-based liver perfusion mapping for evaluating the response of hepatocellular carcinoma to conventional transarterial chemoembolization. J Clin Med. 2021;10:4.
36. Forner A, et al. Current strategy for staging and treatment: the BCLC update and future prospects. Semin Liver Dis. 2010;30(01):061–74.
37. Vogel A, et al. Hepatocellular carcinoma: ESMO clinical practice guidelines for diagnosis, treatment and follow-up†. Ann Oncol. 2018;29(Supplement_4):iv238–55.
38. McVey JC, Sasaki K, Firl DJ. Risk assessment criteria in liver transplantation for hepatocellular carcinoma: proposal to improve transplant oncology. Hepat Oncol. 2020;7(3):HEP26.
39. Cornelis FH, et al. Hepatic arterial embolization using cone beam CT with tumor feeding vessel detection software: impact on hepatocellular carcinoma response. Cardiovasc Intervent Radiol. 2018;41(1):104–11.
40. Joo SM, et al. Optimized performance of flight plan during chemoembolization for hepatocellular carcinoma: importance of the proportion of segmented tumor area. Korean J Radiol. 2016;17(5):771–8.
41. Tamai T, et al. Reduction effect of the quantity of radiation exposure and contrast media by image support system in transarterial chemoembolization for the treatment of hepatocellular carcinoma. J Gastroenterol Hepatol. 2018;33(5):1115–22.
42. Cui Z, et al. A systematic review of automated feeder detection software for locoregional treatment of hepatic tumors. Diagn Interv Imaging. 2020;101(7):439–49.
43. Miyayama S, et al. Outcomes of patients with hepatocellular carcinoma treated with conventional Transarterial chemoembolization using guidance software. J Vasc Interv Radiol. 2019;30(1):10–8.
44. Chiaradia M, et al. Sensitivity and reproducibility of automated feeding artery detection software during Transarterial chemoembolization of hepatocellular carcinoma. J Vasc Interv Radiol. 2018;29(3):425–31.
45. Yao X, et al. Dual-phase cone-beam CT-based navigation imaging significantly enhances tumor detectability and aids superselective transarterial chemoembolization of liver cancer. Acad Radiol. 2018;25(8):1031–7.
46. Soliman MM, et al. Use of virtual injection software to aid in microcatheter positioning during Transarterial chemoembolization. J Vasc Interv Radiol. 2019;30(10):1646–8.
47. Ortiz AK, et al. Injection simulation software identifies missed tumor-supplying vessel in a patient with residual disease after Transarterial chemoembolization for hepatocellular carcinoma. Cardiovasc Intervent Radiol. 2021;44(5):812–4.

6 Conventional TACE (cTACE)

Alberta Cappelli, Rita Golfieri, Violante Mulas, Antonio De Cinque, and Cristina Mosconi

6.1 HCC

6.1.1 *Conventional TACE in* HCC: Technique and Standardised Protocol

6.1.1.1 Haemodynamics in the Liver and HCC

Knowledge of the liver and HCC haemodynamics is important in performing TACE procedures safely and effectively.

In a normal liver, two major branches arise from the terminal hepatic artery: (1) the peribiliary vascular plexus (PBP), which terminates within the portal tract and supplies the bile duct, the portal tract interstitium and the portal vein wall (portal vein vasa vasorum), and (2) an isolated artery, which supplies the liver parenchyma without penetrating the portal vein or bile duct [1].

The majority of the terminal hepatic arterioles connect with the PBP, and blood from the PBP directly drains into the portal venules and hepatic sinusoids.

A possible complication after TACE is bile duct injury, having an incidence that is usually high in the normal liver as compared with the cirrhotic liver due to the greater hypertrophy of the PBP in the cirrhotic liver [2–3].

The refractoriness of a tumour after TACE in the bare area of the liver is due to communication between the isolated artery and the hepatic capsular and arterial plexus, as well as with the extrahepatic arteries, such as the internal mammary and inferior phrenic arteries [4].

Intersegmental collaterals can also develop following TACE promoting tumour recurrence.

In hypervascular HCC, the intranodular arterial supply increases rapidly and the intranodular portal supply decreases gradually; therefore, overt HCC is predominantly supplied by arterial blood [5].

However, some HCCs are still partially supplied by portal blood and by tumours invading the surrounding liver through capsular/extracapsular invasion, mainly located in the periphery of the tumour as well as by microsatellite lesions [6, 7].

Tumour invasion occludes the hepatic veins surrounding HCC so that the tumour blood drains into the peritumoural area through the portal vein remnant in the capsule; this is the feature defined as "corona enhancement" on computed tomography (CT) during hepatic arteriography (CTHA) [8, 9].

A. Cappelli · R. Golfieri (✉) · V. Mulas · C. Mosconi
Department of Radiology, IRCCS Azienda Ospedaliero-Universitaria di Bologna, Bologna, Italy
e-mail: alberta.cappelli@aosp.bo.it; violante.mulas@aosp.bo.it; cristina.mosconi@aosp.bo.it

A. De Cinque
Interventional Neuroradiology Unit, Azienda Ospedaliero-Universitaria di Parma, Parma, Italy
e-mail: adecinque@ao.pr.it

P. Lucatelli (ed.), *Transarterial Chemoembolization (TACE)*,
https://doi.org/10.1007/978-3-031-36261-3_6

6.1.1.2 Conventional TACE (cTACE) Protocol

Conventional TACE (cTACE) was first applied in the early 1980s in Japan and was widely adopted worldwide after evidence of its superiority over the best supportive care for intermediate-stage HCC without PVTT had been proven in two randomised control trials (RCTs) [10, 11]. In these two trials, cTACE consisted of the intra-arterial injection of doxorubicin [10] or cisplatinum [11] mixed with Lipiodol® (Lipiodol® Ultra-Fluid, Guerbet Laboratories, Roissy, France), followed by the administration of an embolic agent.

6.1.1.3 Chemotherapeutic Agents

Treatment is generally based on the intra-arterial injection of a cytotoxic drug, such as an anthracycline (doxorubicin, epirubicin), mitomycin C, cisplatin or idarubicin alone, or a combination of doxorubicin and cisplatin. Chemotherapy drugs are emulsified in the oily radio-opaque agent Lipiodol® and followed by the injection of an embolic agent, such as gelatin sponges (Gelita® Medical), polyvinyl alcohol particles (PVAs) or microspheres in order to induce complete stasis (Fig. 6.1a–d).

Data from the literature have reported that the ideal dose of chemotherapeutic agents should be 10–70 mg for doxorubicin and 10–120 mg for cisplatin per session [12, 13].

There are no standardised criteria to determine the optimal dosage of chemotherapeutic agents; some authors refer to the patient's body surface area (BSA), weight, tumour burden or bilirubin level, and some use a fixed dose. One to three chemotherapeutics are usually used in cTACE, although the value of adding the drug to the embolic agent is still controversial [10, 14–16].

The few RCTs published in the literature have failed to show significant differences in OS between the different drugs (doxorubicin, cisplatin or epirubicin) and different dosages [17–18]. Marelli et al. [12] demonstrated that there was no superiority of any single chemotherapeutic agent over any other agent, or for monodrug chemotherapy versus combination chemotherapy. Some retrospective studies have shown the superiority of cisplatin over doxorubicin/epirubicin in terms of OS [19–21], although a prospective study did not demonstrate any advantage of one over the other [22]. Moreover, cisplatin may induce renal toxicity, thrombocytopenia, hepatic failure and hypersensitivity reactions, generally having an increased risk based on the number of treatments [23].

Miriplatin is a lipophilic platinum chemotherapeutic that is available only in Japan [24]. Nowadays, miriplatin is mainly used in balloon-occluded TACE due to its association with less arterial damage [25].

No adequate scientific evidence has been reported regarding the value of switching the chemotherapeutics in HCC nonresponders back to the initial form of cTACE [22, 24, 26].

Lipiodol® (Lipiodol® Ultra-Fluid, Guerbet Laboratories, Roissy, France) is an iodinated ethyl ester of poppy seed oil, first used as oily contrast medium for lymphangiographic studies. It was used for the first time in 1974 [27] and became popular in the early 1980s with the increased use of cTACE. Lipiodol® was introduced as a drug carrier [28–30]. Thanks to its ability to remain inside the tumour for a long period of time [30] and therefore to enhance the anti-tumoural effects of the drug. Lipiodol® has a preferential accumulation and longer retention in the target hypervascularised lesions rather than in the normal liver, and selectively remains in tumour nodules for several weeks to over a year.

In the normal liver parenchyma, Lipiodol® accumulates in the portal venules using arterioportal shunts, and it is gradually released into the systemic circulation via the hepatic sinusoids or undergoes phagocytosis by Kupffer cells [29, 30]. The absence of Kupffer cells inside the hypervascularised tumours enhances the so-called siphoning effect, resulting in embolic effects on smaller vessels [31].

Moreover, Lipiodol® circulates beyond the tumour-feeding arteries into the distal portal branches through the peribiliary capillary plexus and the drainage route, resulting in a temporary embolic effect on both the hepatic artery and the portal branches [30, 32–34]. The ability of

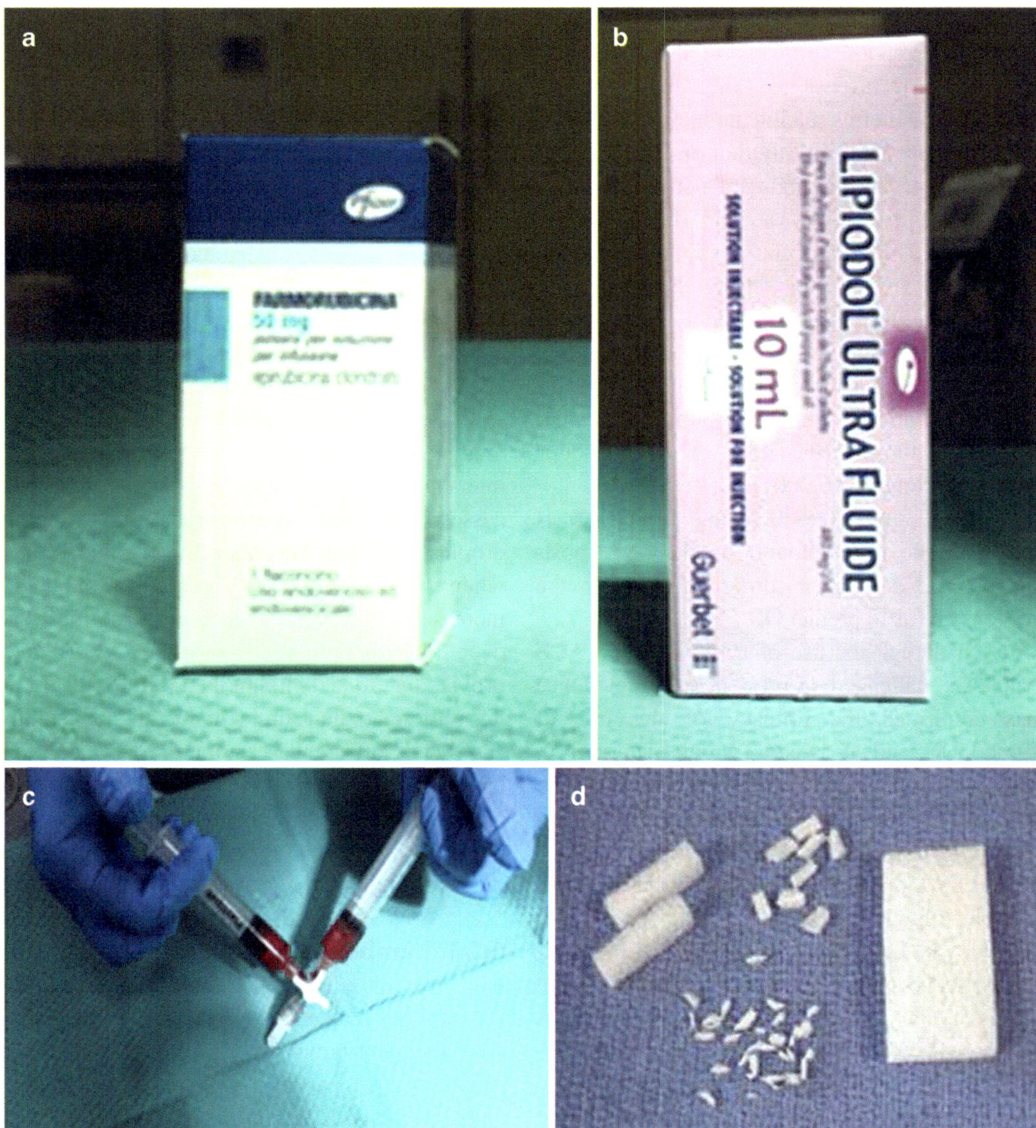

Fig. 6.1 cTACE protocol and therapeutic agents. (**a**) Farmorubicin® and (**b**) Lipiodol® packages. (**c**) Image showing the emulsion of the chemotherapeutic with Lipiodol®. (**d**) Embolic agents. Sponge (Gelita® Medical). *Abbreviations:* cTACE, conventional transarterial chemoembolisation

iodised oil to pass through the arterial communication network and the neighbouring hepatic arterial branches and/or extrahepatic arteries allows identifying the occult feeding arteries and may prevent the arterial collateral supply to the tumour [35, 36].

The maximum dose of Lipiodol recommended for one cTACE procedure is generally 10 mL in Japan and 15 mL in Western countries [37].

Another major advantage of Lipiodol® is its radio-opacity that makes it capable of being visualised in the vascular bed during treatment in order to control the delivery of the treatment by continuous visualisation of the therapeutic agents until the tumour vascular bed is saturated and stasis is obtained in the most peripheral branches. Miyayama et al. [7] demonstrated that visualisation of the small peripheral portal branches around the tumour with Lipiodol® is a predictive factor for tumour response to treatment and for a lower rate of local recurrence and complete necrosis of the tumour and of its satellite nodules.

Miyayama [34] recently demonstrated a relationship between the grades of portal vein visualisation with Lipiodol® and local tumour recurrence. The authors classified three grades of portal vein visualisation during the procedure: grade 0, no visualisation; grade 1, visualisation adjacent to the tumour and grade 2, visualisation in the entire area target, reporting local recurrence rates in the grade 2 group significantly lower than those in the grades 1 and 0 groups ($p < 0.0485$ and $p < 0.0001$, respectively).

Another advantage of using Lipiodol® is detecting the intratumoural uptake on a post-procedure CT scan in order to evaluate the response so as to predict OS.

Even though the use of Lipiodol® in TACE has been challenged, at present, strong evidence has confirmed the efficacy of the use of Lipiodol®, and it is still widely adopted in cTACE protocols [12].

Two types of iodised oil emulsion can be prepared: water-in-oil emulsion (WOE) and oil-in-water emulsion (OWE). The former has stronger embolic effects than the latter [38].

Kiyoyuki et al. [39] have evaluated the ischemic effects of arterial embolisation between two different embolic agents: 75 μm microspheres and pure WOE. The authors found significant differences in the percentage of the necrotic areas in the tumour and the complete response (CR) ratio between the two groups. The mean percentage of the necrotic ratios were 99.9% in the WOE group and 87.6% in the microsphere group. Furthermore, the necrotic ratio in the WOE group was significantly higher than that in the microsphere group ($p = 0.029$). The CR rate in the WOE group was significantly higher than that in the microsphere group ($p = 0.041$). The WOE showed stronger anti-tumoural effects, thanks to its ability to occlude both the tumour-feeding artery and the portal vein.

In general, preparation of the cTACE mixture involves two different modalities, either the WOE technique, which consists of using the chemotherapeutic agent diluted with an aqueous solution (or contrast media) and then mixed with Lipiodol®, or the chemotherapeutic-in-oil (CiO) technique in which the final emulsion contains the drug mixed directly in Lipiodol® [38, 40]. To better standardise the procedure, some points should be clarified: what happens when the number of mixes changes, what happens to the emulsions over time and what are the intra- and inter-operator variabilities in the preparation of emulsions using different methods. Renzulli et al. [41] investigated the chemical and physical characteristics, and the behaviour over time of emulsions for cTACE, and assessed intra- and inter-operator variabilities in the preparation processes. The authors demonstrated that the mean droplet diameter decreased non-significantly when the number of pumping exchanges increased; however, it increased significantly over time for both WOE and CiO. It was well proven that after remixing the mixture, the droplets returned to their initial diameters without any significant differences in the intra- and inter-operator variabilities ($P > 0.01$). The study concluded that any interventional radiologist, regardless of their experience, can prepare these mixtures, making the procedure standardisable.

6.1.1.4 Embolic Agents

No consensus exists regarding the most appropriate embolic agents. In general, the optimal embolic agent (among gelatin sponges (Gelita® Medical), PVA particles and microspheres, steel coils, autologous blood clots and degradable starch microspheres) depends on its ability to embolise the peripheral arteries as much as possible to both stop the hepatic arterial flow and to prevent the development of collateral feeding vessels to the tumour. Gelatin sponges are the most widely used embolic agent in cTACE; they have the advantage of inducing temporary occlusion, making sequential treatment possible [42]. By adding arterial occlusion with gelatin sponges after the injection of Lipiodol®, both the hepatic artery and the portal vein are embolised, leading to potential liver damage. Therefore, selective catheterisation is mandatory in order to minimise liver toxicity during cTACE.

6.2 Conventional TACE (cTACE) Technique: Superselective TACE

6.2.1 Limitation of TACE and Necessity for Curative TACE

As a consequence of what has been described above, there are two possible causes of local tumour recurrence after TACE, namely:

1. *The portal blood supply to HCC* via the portal venules and hepatic sinusoids induced by the inversion of the portal flow due to the blockage of the arterial flow.
2. *The arterial collateral supply to HCC* from the extrahepatic arteries by means of communication between the hepatic capsular arterial plexus and the isolated artery described above.

In order to be curative, the above two factors can be acted upon to reduce the local tumour recurrence after TACE.

It has been well demonstrated that a CR after the initial TACE is the most robust predictor of long-term survival [43].

A non-effective TACE frequently induces a change in the tumour, making it more aggressive, i.e., a sarcomatous appearance or a mixed hepatocholangiocellular phenotype [44, 45].

Moreover, the hypoxia induced by TACE stimulates the vascular endothelial growth factor (VEGF) production by the residual tumour cells that, in turn, could promote tumour progression [46, 47].

As a consequence, it is mandatory to occlude each tumour feeder; as a general rule, the main tumour-feeding artery should be embolised at the end of the procedure since the retention of iodised oil and contrast material may hide other small feeders. Moreover, the embolic agents may flow back through the minor feeding arteries [48].

Another fundamental rule is to first embolise the feeding branch of the extrahepatic artery when present since the extrahepatic arterial blood flow immediately increases when the hepatic arterial flow is occluded [49].

Concerning cTACE, Yamakado et al. [50] have also reported that technique has an impact on patient survival. In HCC patients with nodules ≤7 cm and with ≤5 lesions, the prognosis of patients who underwent selective/superselective cTACE was significantly better than that of patients treated with non-selective cTACE ($p = 0.033$).

As a consequence, superselective cTACE is strongly recommended for patients with Child-Pugh scores of 5–8 and HCC nodules ≤7 cm and with ≤5 lesions.

On the other hand, for tumours >7 cm but with ≤3 lesions, stepwise superselective cTACE is also performed with a curative purpose [48, 51].

The authors reported a 5-year survival rate of 23.1% in large HCCs >10 cm (mean, 130 ± 27.6 mm [range, 101–193], single nodule [n = 12], 2–9 nodules [n = 6, mean, 4.2 ± 2.6] and 10 nodules [n = 7, including 2 with 50 tumours], with vascular invasion [n = 5]) and of 38.9% with <3 lesions; cTACE of the extrahepatic collateral arteries was required in 84% of patients.

Another possible option could be a bland embolisation with gelatin sponge particles followed by cTACE for large HCCs in order to safely embolise the tumour [52]. This indicates that cTACE is also effective for localised large HCCs (Fig. 6.2a–h).

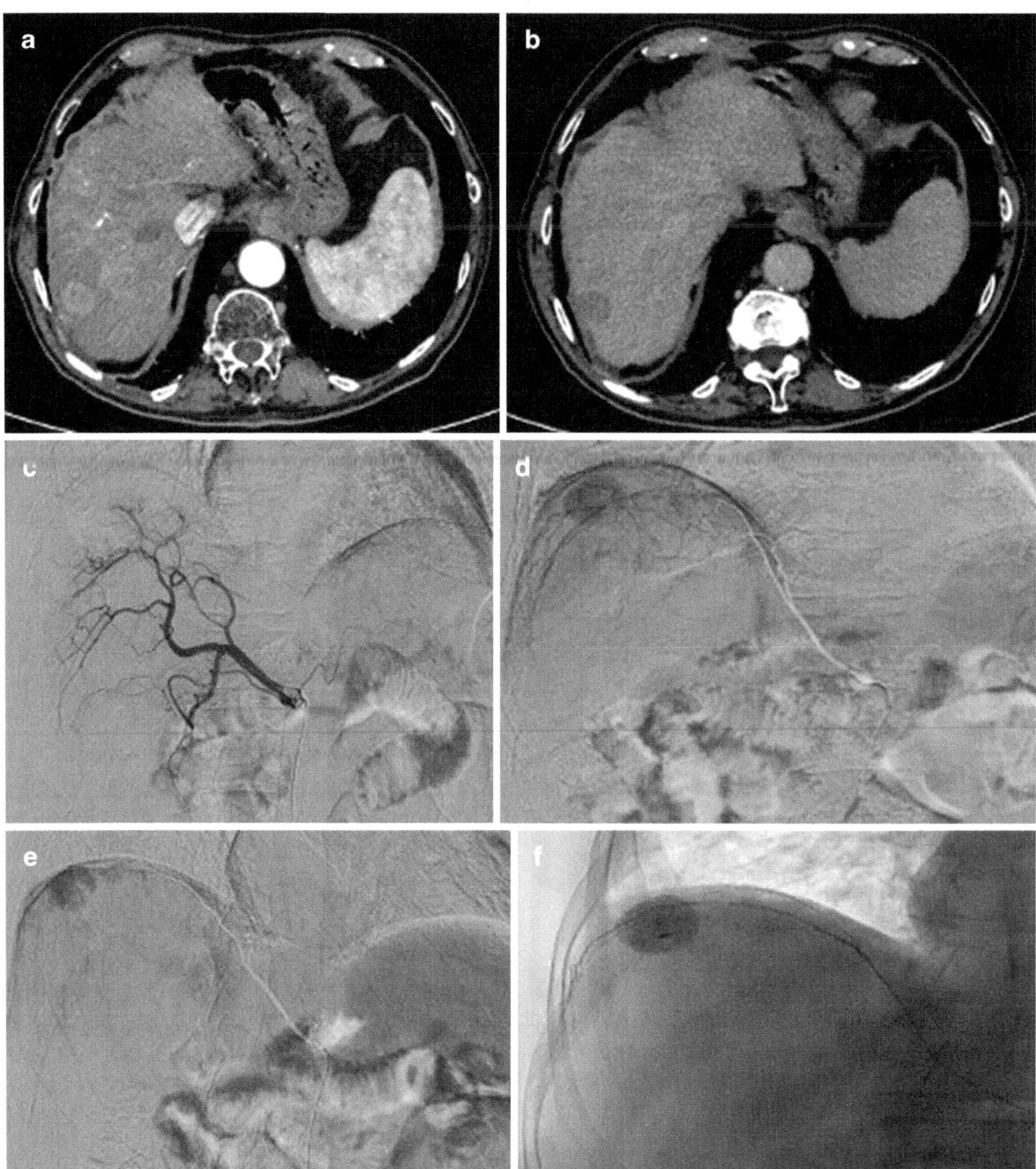

Fig. 6.2 (**a**, **b**) Pretreatment CT: a 20-mm HCC is seen in segment VII, highly hypervascular in the arterial phase (**a**) and rapid washout in the portal phase (**b**). (**c**) Pretreatment angiogram showing no visualisation of the nodule from the proper hepatic artery. (**d**) The angiogram performed in the right inferior phrenic artery showing the main feeding artery contributing to perfusion of the nodule. (**e–f**) Images showing the selective angiographic study performed in the distal vessel of the inferior phrenic artery after chemotherapy mixture injection showing (**f**) complete stasis of the arterial flow through the vessels feeding the nodule, maintaining the flow into the proximal trunk of the phrenic artery. (**g, h**) Axial (**g**) and coronal MPR (**h**) cone-beam CT angiogram showing the superselective uptake of the Lipiodol® by the target HCC. *Abbreviations: CT* computed tomography; *HCC* hepatocellular carcinoma; *MPR* multiplanar reformation

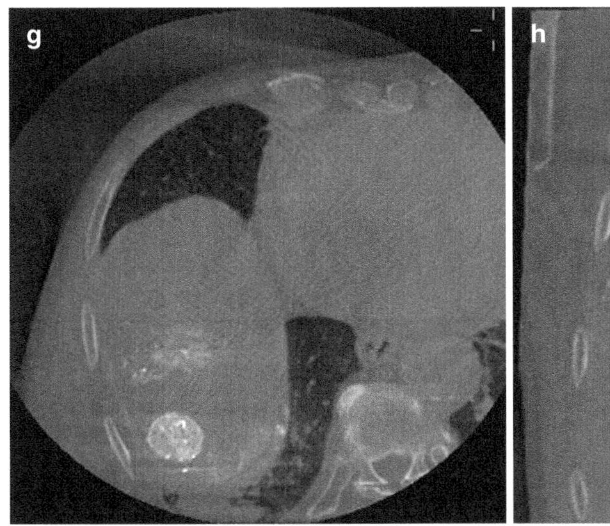

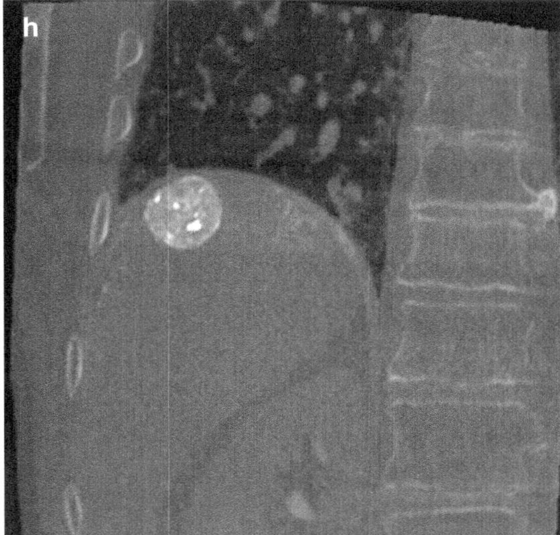

Fig. 6.2 (continued)

6.3 Conventional TACE in Intrahepatic Cholangiocarcinoma (ICC)

Intrahepatic cholangiocarcinoma (ICC) is a relatively rare biliary adenocarcinoma; however. Its incidence rate has significantly increased over the last several decades and accounts for 10–20% of all primary liver cancers [53].

The prognosis of patients has also changed, thanks to the advanced diagnostic and treatment approach to this disease. Surgical intervention is possible at the time of diagnosis in approximately 54–70% of patients [53, 54]. The prognosis for these patients is poor with a reported median survival of 5–8 months.

While incidence is increasing and more risk factors are being discovered, additional effort is needed to improve outcomes of this unfortunate disease.

Management strategies include multidisciplinary treatments, taking into account new drugs for systemic chemotherapy and targeted intra-arterial and surgical therapies. Liver transplantation is becoming a therapeutic option in certain selected cases.

Systemic chemotherapy traditionally has a poor response, and a variety of intra-arterial therapies (IATs) have been explored.

Therefore, the role of IAT is increasingly being investigated in ICC patients.

Referrals to centres of excellence and enrolment in novel clinical trials are recommended for patients with unresectable or recurrent ICC.

This chapter discusses the role of cTACE in the treatment of ICC.

6.3.1 Background

Conventional TACE is the most commonly used intra-arterial technique for unresectable ICC. The protocol is the same as for other cancers, and due to the main central location of ICC within the liver, angiographic evaluation of both the right and the left hepatic arteries is required to ensure selective treatment of the tumour-feeding vessels (Fig. 6.3a–e). The most commonly used drug combination consists of doxorubicin, cisplatin and mitomycin C; however, gemcitabine has also been used [55, 56]. In general, cTACE is well tolerated by the patients, and no major adverse events have been reported.

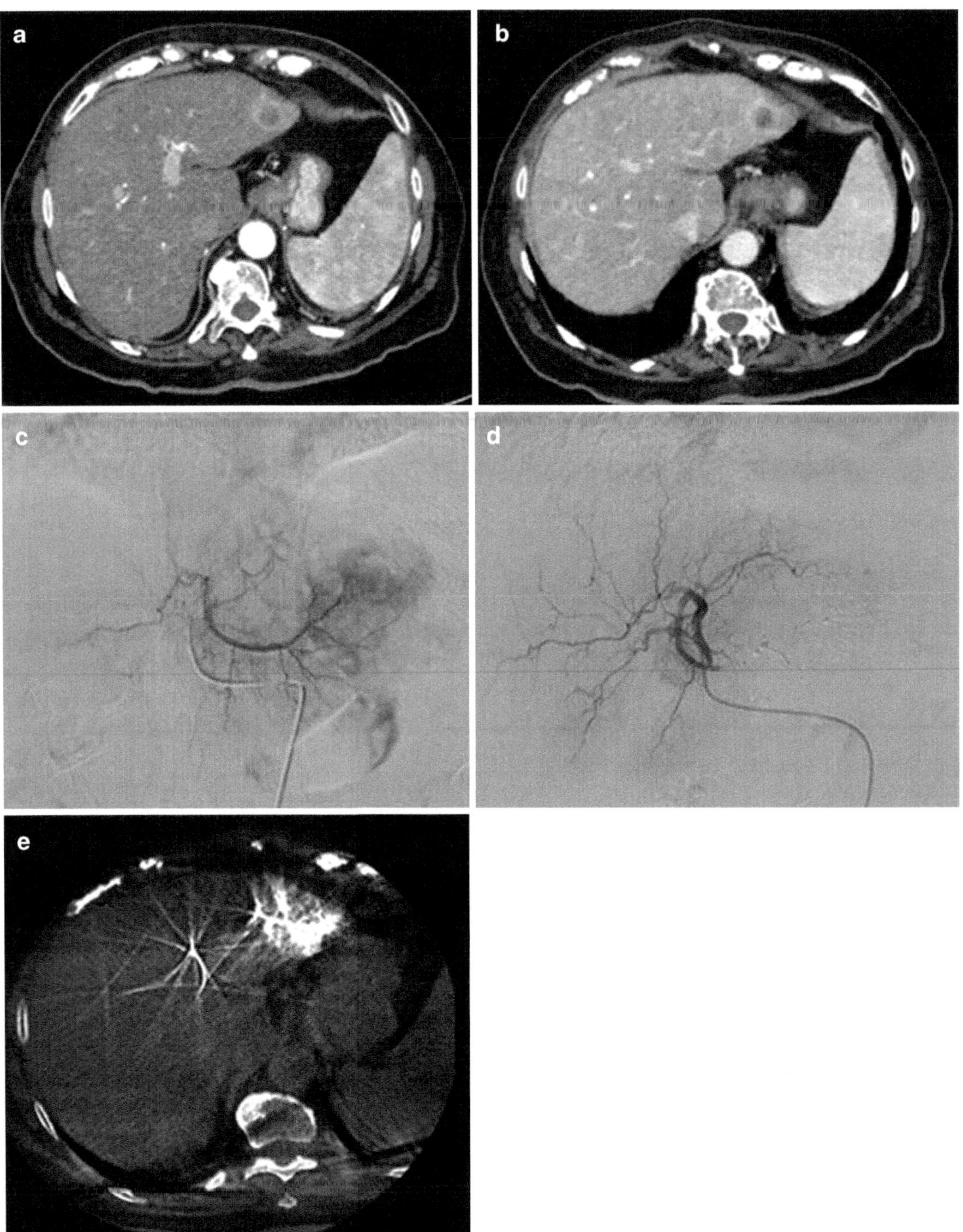

Fig. 6.3 (**a, b**) Pretreatment CT: a single nodule of ICC is seen in the left lobe with peripheral enhancement in the arterial phase and necrotic central area (**a**) and progressive filling in the portal phase (**b**). (**c**) Pretreatment angiogram showing nodule feeding from the left distal hepatic artery. (**d**) The angiogram performed after superselective cTACE showing the complete segmentary exclusion of the target lesion from the vascularisation. (**e**) Axial cone-beam CT angiogram showing the superselective uptake of the Lipiodol® into the target ICC

6.3.2 Clinical Evidence and Tumour Response

Few prospective studies have investigated the clinical outcomes in ICC treated with cTACE; the majority of the retrospective studies did not use a standardised procedure protocol. However, data from the literature have reported a potential survival benefit, a median OS of 9.1 months, in patients with unresectable ICC [57, 58]. Moreover, the combination of gemcitabine and cisplatin has been reported to have shown better survival than gemcitabine alone (13.8 vs. 6.3 months, $P < 0.001$). Another chemotherapeutic agent commonly used for cTACE is mitomycin C; in a retrospective survival analysis that involved 15 patients, the median OS was 16.3 months (95% CI, 9.4–32.5 months) [59].

A more recent retrospective study analysed the survival benefits among all available therapeutic options for ICC. About 32 (11.7%) out of 273 patients with ICC without extrahepatic disease underwent TACE with mitomycin C ($n = 29$) or doxorubicin-eluting beads ($n = 3$). The median OS was 11 months as compared to 28 months of the surgical patients; however, it should be noted that there were significant variations in the median OS of patients with positive lymph node status (N1; 9 months) or a positive resection margin (R+; 11 months). The authors concluded that surgery did not show a significant survival benefit for those patients with R+ or N1 as compared to those treated with TACE [60].

Another study carried out by Park et al. [61] compared cTACE in 72 unresectable ICC patients with 83 patients undergoing symptomatic supportive therapy. The median OS in the TACE group was significantly better than that in the supportive therapy group (12.2 months vs. 3.3 months, respectively, $P < 0.001$). Moreover, according to the RECIST criteria, patients who were *responders* to TACE reported a significantly higher median OS as compared to those who were *nonresponders* (22 months vs. 10.9 months, respectively, $P = 0.0001$).

Regarding the use of cTACE with different drug combinations as an adjuvant therapy after radical surgery, the median OS in the adjuvant cTACE group was 12 months as compared to 5 months in the only surgery group, even though cTACE did not delay the recurrence of the disease [62].

More recently, Yang et al. [63] investigated the combination of TACE with microwave ablation therapy in 26 patients with advanced ICC.

The authors reported a complete ablation in 36 out of 39 lesions (92.3%) without major complications, and a reported median OS of 19.5 months and a PFS of 6.2 months (range, 3–12 months).

Therefore, combination therapy should be considered to be a safe and feasible alternative, even though no matched pair analysis with a control group was carried out.

Regarding the few available prospective trials, in 2012, Vogl et al. [64] reported a median OS of 13 months in 115 patients with unresectable ICC who had undergone cTACE from the first treatment without differences in the drug regimens.

Other studies have reported a median OS ranging from 20 to 23 months from the time of diagnosis and almost 15 months from the first cTACE. Patients with prior chemotherapy had significantly prolonged survival as compared to those who had received cTACE only [65, 66].

When comparing TACE with Yittrium-90 radioembolisation (Y90-RE) and RFA in 55 patients with unresectable ICC and a good PS (median ECOG 1), as regards local tumour control, TACE had the best tumour response for progressive disease (PD) and Y90-RE had the best PR. The median OS of all patients was 16 months from first treatment and 33.1 months from diagnosis [67].

Yittrium-90 radioembolisation was, for the most part, performed in multinodular disease whereas TACE was performed in single lesions without PVTT. The most aggressive ICCs required additional systemic chemotherapy.

One of the independent factors influencing OS was the objective tumour response (liver only) with almost 30 months for CR and PR, and 9.3 months for stable disease (SD) and PD ($P = 0.005$). Ongoing prospective studies include

Table 6.1 Current level of evidence for the treatment of intrahepatic cholangiocarcinoma with conventional transcatheter arterial chemoembolisation (cTACE). *Abbreviations: OS* overall survival; *mo.* months; *N/A* not available

Author	Patients	Line of therapy	Drug agent used	Embolic agent used	ORR	PFS (months)	OS (months)
Hunt (1990)	19	FL	FU	DSM	n.r.	n.r.	13
Sanz Altamira (1997)	40	FL	FU, MITO	Ethiodized oil, Gelfoam	n.r.	n.r.	10
Tellez (1998)	30	SL	CDDP, DOXO, MITO	Gelfoam	63	n.r.	8.6
Bavisotto (1999)	20	SL	CDDP	PVA	70	4.2	14.3
Salman (2002)	24	SL	FU	PVA	20.8	n.r.	11
Hong (2009)	21	SL	CDDP, DOXO, MITO	PVA	n.r.	n.r.	7.7
Vogl (2009)	463	STL	MITO, GEM, IRI	Ethiodized oil, DSM	14.7	n.r.	13
Albert (2011)	121	SL	CDDP, DOXO, MITO	Ethiodized oil, PVA	43	5	11
Nishiofuku (2021)	24	SL	CDDP, DOXO, MITO	Ethiodized oil, PVA, DSM	61.1	8.8	8.8

the first RCTs that compare the efficacy of Y90-RE and cTACE in terms of radiological response [68, 69].

However, the treatment protocols, timing and drug regimens in all of these studies are extremely different, making the cTACE procedure in the setting of ICC non-standardisable.

Table 6.1 reports the current level of evidence for treating ICC with cTACE.

6.3.3 Conventional TACE in Liver Metastases

6.3.3.1 From Colorectal Tumours (CRLM)

Colorectal cancer is the third most common cancer in terms of incidence and the second leading cause of death worldwide with an estimated 881,000 deaths in 2018 [70–73].

Adenocarcinomas are the most common type of small bowel cancer and account for approximately 3% of all digestive system cancers. Approximately 10,590 cases are expected to have been diagnosed in 2019 [74].

This explains why innovative treatments for colorectal liver metastases (CRLM) have been extensively studied. The standard for radical treatment is surgical resection combined with systemic chemotherapy.

However, only approximately 25% of patients are amenable to resection at diagnosis [75]; up to 80% of patients develop liver recurrence up to 10 years post-surgery, the majority of them within the first 2 years after surgery [76].

Therefore, in the setting of unresectable disease or potentially resectable disease, other approaches have been developed in order to control the disease, to treat recurrences and to prolong patient survival.

In addition to the percutaneous procedures such as radiofrequency ablation and microwaves, intra-arterial techniques, such as cTACE, DEB-TACE, transarterial embolisation (TAE), Y90-RE and hepatic arterial infusion chemotherapy (HAIC), have been widely applied by multidisciplinary teams.

These therapies are generally indicated for patients with oligometastatic disease, who are not suitable for surgery or other curative locoregional therapies, or without any response, disease progression or toxicity/contraindication to systemic chemotherapy.

While TACE is well established as a therapy in the setting of HCC patients, its role in the treatment of CRLM is more limited. Doxorubicin, cisplatin and mitomycin C are the common chemotherapeutic agents used in TACE for the treatment of CRLM.

However, data from the literature have reported a great variety of treatment protocols with different combinations of chemotherapeutic agents, microspheres and embolic agents used alone or in combination, including lipiodol oil, collagen particles, PVA particles or trisacryl gelatin microspheres [77]. Data from prospective studies [78] have reported 2-year survival rates of 66% and a CR of 10%. Two older studies [79, 80] have shown median survival ranging from 8.6 to 10 months with a median duration of response of 7 months.

In these studies, it has been well established that patients with large tumour burdens (75% of the liver volume) may not benefit from this procedure.

Vogl et al. [78] have reported the results of 463 patients treated with cTACE that included mitomycin C alone, mitomycin C with gemcitabine or mitomycin C with irinotecan followed by microsphere embolisation.

The 1- and 2-year survival rates were 62% and 28%, respectively, without significant differences between cTACE regimens.

Other authors [81] have reported the results of TACE with cisplatin, doxorubicin, mitomycin C and Lipiodol mixture followed by PVA particles in 121 patients (245 treatments), showing a median time-to-disease progression (TTP) of 5 months and a median survival of 33 months from initial diagnosis and 9 months from the first treatment.

As expected, OS was significantly better when TACE treatment was performed after first- or second-line systemic therapy than after more lines of chemotherapy (Table 6.2).

It is currently considered to be a good therapeutic approach for patients with colorectal cancer and liver-limited disease who fail the available chemotherapeutic options [82–87].

In conclusion, even though there is no high-level clinical evidence to applying TACE treatment in CRLM, intra-arterial treatments allowed the authors to tailor their clinical approach to the individual based on disease status and clinical condition.

Additional RCTs are needed to better define the role and the timing of these therapies in combination with surgery and standard systemic therapy.

6.3.3.2 From Neuroendocrine Tumours (NETs)

Transarterial chemoembolisation/TAE are generally indicated in cases of nonresectable and clinically symptomatic metastatic NETs due to hormone production or bulky multifocal disease. In this setting of patients, surgery and percutaneous ablative therapies are not suitable. Even though somatostatin agents induce an initial control of symptoms, TACE can result in durable elimination of hormonal symptoms [88]. However, many patients with hormonally active liver metastases also have extrahepatic disease; thus, hormonal treatment should not be withheld after TACE. Moreover, TACE/TAE may also be used in cases where there is a large burden of liver disease in the absence of clinical symptoms. Median survival time ranges from 39.6 to 80 months, and symptoms resolve in 60–90% of cases [89].

6.3.3.3 From Other Types of Tumours

Metastatic Uveal Melanoma. Tumour response after cisplatin, fotemustine or bis-chloroethyl-nitrosourea cTACE ranges from 6 to 39%, and median OS does not exceed 10 months [90–93].

However, patients defined as *responders* to TACE have a longer OS than *nonresponders* (15–22 months vs. 5–9 months). Furthermore, the extent of liver replacement affects median OS:

Table 6.2 Summary of results from key studies adopting conventional TACE in the treatment of unresectable liver metastases from colorectal cancer

	Study Design	Drug agent (TACE)	Control groups	Study cohort (n)	ECOG status	*Extrahepatic lesion*	Previous systemic chemotherapy	Adverse events (grade III/IV)	Median OS (mo from first cTACE)
Gusani et al. (2008)	Retrospective	Gemcitabine, cisplatin, oxaliplatin	No	42	0–1	$n = 19$ (45%)	N/A	Myocardial infarction ($n = 1$), hepatic abscess ($n = 1$), hyperbilirubinemia ($n = 2$), thrombocytopenia ($n = 2$)	9.1
Herber et al. (2007)	Retrospective	Mitomycin-c	No	15	N/A	N/A	$n = 4$ (27%)	Anaphylactic shock (7%), gastric ulceration (7%)	16.3
Scheuermann et al. (2013)	Retrospective	Mitomycin-c	cTACE (n = 32) vs surgery (n = 130) vs systemic chemotherapy (n = 111)	273	N/A	No	N/A	Massive ascites ($n = 1$), dissection or occlusion of the hepatic artery ($n = 2$)	11
Park et al. (2011)	Retrospective	Cisplatin	cTACE (n = 32) vs supportive care (n = 83)	155	0–2	$N = 39$ (54%) in no TACE group; $n = 50$ (60%) in supportive care group	No	Hematological toxicity events ($n = 9$, 13%), non hematological toxicity events ($n = 17$, 24%),	12.2
Shen et al. (2011)	Retrospective	Adjuvant 5-FU, epirubicin, hydrocamptothecin, gemcitabine Carboplatin	Hepatic resction only (n = 72) vs adjuvant cTACE (n = 53)	125	0–1	No	No	No	12
Yang et al. (2015)	Retrospective	Gemcitabine, oxaliplatin, (cTACE no in combination with microwave ablation)	No	26	0–2	No	No	No	19.5
Vogl et al. (2012)	Prospective	Gemcitabine, mitomycin-c, cisplain	No	115	N/A	N/A	N/A	No	13

	Study Design	Drug agent (TACE)	Control groups	Study cohort (n)	ECOG status	*Extrahepatic lesion*	Previous systemic chemotherapy	Adverse events (grade III/IV)	Median OS (mo from first cTACE)
Burger et al. (2005)	Prospective	Doxorubicine, cisplatin, mitomycin-c	No	17	0–3	$n = 5$ (29%)	$n = 6$ (35%)	Treatment related mortality (6%), acute cholecystitis $n = 1$ (6%), ascites $n = 1$ (6%)	N/A (23 from diagnosis)
Kiefer et al. (2011)	Prospective	Doxorubicine, cisplatin, mitomycin-c	No	62	0–2	$n = 19$ (31%)	$n = 18$ (29%)	Pulmonary edema and elevated cardiac enzymes ($n = 1$) Pulmonary infarct ($n = 1$), severe postembolization syndrome ($n = 1$) Hyperglycaemia ($n = 1$), acute renal failure and dehydration postprocedure ($n = 1$),	15

- < 25%, 14–17 months
- 25–50%, 5–6 months
- 50–75%, 5–7.3 months
- > 75%, 2.1–5.6 months [89–95].

In a retrospective review of 53 patients treated with immunoembolisation or bis-chloroethyl-nitrosourea cTACE, immunoembolisation showed significantly longer median OS (20.4 months vs. 9.8 months) and better systemic PFS (12.4 months vs. 4.8 months) [96]. Additional studies are needed regarding this type of metastatic lesion.

Other Liver Metastases Soft tissue sarcomas, such as gastrointestinal stromal tumours, breast carcinoma and gynaecologic tumours, have been successfully treated with TACE. Overall survival seems to be improved as compared with the control group [97–100]. However, RCTs are needed to better evaluate the clinical outcomes in this setting of metastatic patients.

References

1. Ekataksin W. The isolated artery: an intrahepatic arterial pathway that can bypass the lobular parenchyma in mammalian livers. Hepatology. 2000;31:269–79.
2. Kobayashi S, Nakanuma Y, Terada T, Matsui O. Postmortem survey of bile duct necrosis and biloma in hepatocellular carcinoma after transcatheter arterial chemoembolization therapy: relevance to microvascular damages of peribiliary capillary plexus. Am J Gastroenterol. 1993;88:1410–5.
3. Kobayashi S, Nakamuma Y, Matsui O. Histopathology of portal tracts in livers after transcatheter arterial chemo-embolization therapy for hepatocellular carcinoma. J Gastroenterol Hepatol. 1994;9:45–54.
4. Yoshida K, Matsui O, Miyayama S, Ibukuro K, Yoneda N, Inoue D, Kozaka K, Minami T, Koda W, Gabata T. Isolated arteries originating from the intrahepatic arteries: anatomy, function, and importance in intervention. J Vasc Interv Radiol. 2018;29:531–537.e1.
5. Hayashi M, Matsui O, Ueda K, Kawamori Y, Kadoya M, Yoshikawa J, Gabata T, Takashima T, Nonomua A, Nakanuma Y. Correlation between the blood supply and grade of malignancy of hepatocellular nodules associated with liver cirrhosis: evaluation by CT during intraarterial injection of contrast medium. AJR Am J Roentgenol. 1999;172:969–76.
6. Kuroda C, Sakurai M, Monden M, Marukawa T, Hosoki T, Tokunaga K, Wakasa K, Okamura J, Kozuka T. Limitation of transcatheter arterial chemoembolization using iodized oil for small hepatocellular carcinoma. A study in resected cases. Cancer. 1991;67:81–6.
7. Miyayama S. Treatment strategy of Transarterial chemoembolization for hepatocellular carcinoma. Appl Sci. 2020;10(7337):3–19.
8. Kitao A, Zen Y, Matsui O, Gabata T, Nakanuma Y. Hepatocarcinogenesis: multistep changes of drainage vessels at CT during arterial portography and hepatic arteriography–radiologic-pathologic correlation. Radiology. 2009;252:605–14.
9. Ueda K, Matsui O, Kawamori Y, Nakamuma Y, Kadoya M, Yoshikawa J, Gabata T, Nonomura A, Takashima T. Hypervascular hepatocellular carcinoma: evaluation of hemodynamics with dynamic CT during hepatic arteriography. Radiology. 1998;206:161–6.
10. Llovet JM, Real MI, Montaña X, Planas R, Coll S, Aponte J, Ayuso C, Sala M, Muchart J, Solà R, Rodés J, Bruix J, Barcelona Liver Cancer Group. Arterial embolisation or chemoembolisation versus symptomatic treatment in patients with unresectable hepatocellular carcinoma: a randomised controlled trial. Lancet. 2002;359(9319):1734–9.
11. Lo CM, Ngan H, Tso WK, Liu CL, Lam CM, Poon RT, Fan ST, Wong J. Randomized controlled trial of transarterial lipiodol chemoembolization for unresectable hepatocellular carcinoma. Hepatology. 2002;35(5):1164–71.
12. Marelli L, Stigliano R, Triantos C, Senzolo M, Cholongitas E, Davies N, et al. Transarterial therapy for hepatocellular carcinoma: which technique is more effective? A systematic review of cohort and randomized studies. Cardiovasc Intervent Radiol. 2007;30:6–25.
13. Bruix J, Sala M, Llovet JM. Chemoembolization for hepatocellular carcinoma. Gastroenterology. 2004;127:S179–88.
14. Cammà C, Schepis F, Orlando A, Albanese M, Shahied L, Trevisani F, Andreone P, Craxì A, Cottone M. Transarterial chemoembolization for unresectable hepatocellular carcinoma: meta-analysis of randomized controlled trials. Radiology. 2002;224:47–54.
15. Malagari K, Pomoni M, Kelekis A, Pomoni A, Dourakis S, Spyridopoulos T, Moschouris H, Emmanouil E, Rizos S, Kelekis D. Prospective randomized comparison of chemoembolization with doxorubicin-eluting beads and bland embolization with BeadBlock for hepatocellular carcinoma. Cardiovasc Intervent Radiol. 2010 Jun;33(3):541–51.
16. Brown KT, Do RK, Gonen M, Covey AM, Getrajdman GI, Sofocleous CT, Jarnagin WR, D'Angelica MI, Allen PJ, Erinjeri JP, et al. Randomized trial of hepatic artery embolization for hepatocellular carcinoma using doxorubicin-eluting

microspheres compared with embolization with microspheres alone. J Clin Oncol. 2016;34:2046–53.
17. Kawai S, Tani M, Okamura J, Ogawa M, Ohashi Y, Monden M, et al. Prospective and randomized trial of Lipiodol-transcatheter arterial chemoemboliza-tion for treatment of hepatocellular carcinoma: a comparison of epirubicin and doxorubicin (second cooperative study). The Cooperative Study Group for Liver Cancer Treatment of Japan. Semin Oncol. 1997;24:S6-38–45.
18. Watanabe S, Nishioka M, Ohta Y, Ogawa N, Ito S, Yamamoto Y. Prospective and randomized controlled study of chemoembolization therapy in patients with advanced hepatocellular carci-noma. Cooperative Study Group for Liver Cancer Treatment in Shikoku area. Cancer Chemother Pharmacol. 1994;33:S93–6.
19. Kamada K, Nakanishi T, Kitamoto M, Aikata H, Kawakami Y, Ito K, Kajiyama G. Long-term prog-nosis of patients undergoing transcatheter arterial chemoembolization for unresectable hepatocellular carcinoma: comparison of cisplatin lipiodol suspen-sion and doxorubicin hydrochloride emulsion. J Vasc Interv Radiol. 2001;12:847–54.
20. Yodono H, Matsuo K, Shinohara A. A retrospective comparative study of epirubicin-lipiodol emulsion and cisplatin-lipiodol suspension for use with trans-catheter arterial chemoembolization. Anti-Cancer Drugs. 2011;22:277–82.
21. Kasai K, Ushio A, Sawara K, Miyamoto Y, Kasai Y, Oikawa K, Kuroda H, Takikawa Y, Suzuki K. Transcatheter arterial chemoembolization with a fine-powder formulation of cisplatin for hepa-tocellular carcinoma. World J Gastroenterol. 2010;16:3437–44.
22. Sahara S, Kawai N, Sato M, Minamiguchi H, Nakai M, Takasaka I, Nakata K, Ikoma A, Sawa N, Sonomura T, et al. Prospective comparison of trans-catheter arterial chemoembolization with Lipiodol-epirubicin and Lipiodol-cisplatin for treatment of recurrent hepatocellular carcinoma. Jpn J Radiol. 2010;28:362–8.
23. Kawaoka T, Aikata H, Katamura Y, Takaki S, Waki K, Hiramatsu A, Takahashi S, Hieda M, Kakizawa H, Chayama K. Hypersensitivity reactions to trans-catheter chemoembolization with cisplatin and Lipiodol suspension for unresectable hepatocellular carcinoma. J Vasc Interv Radiol. 2010;21:1219–25.
24. Ikeda M, Kudo M, Aikata H, Nagamatsu H, Ishii H, Yokosuka O, Torimura T, Morimoto M, Ikeda K, Kumada H, et al. Transarterial chemoembolization with miriplatin vs. epirubicin for unresectable hepa-tocellular carcinoma: a phase III randomized trial. J Gastroenterol. 2018;53:281–90.
25. Irie T, Kuramochi M, Takahashi N. Dense accumu-lation of Lipiodol emulsion in hepatocellular car-cinoma nodule during selective balloon-occluded transarterial chemoembolization: measurement of balloon occluded arterial stump pressure. Cardiovasc Intervent Radiol. 2013;36:706–13.
26. Maeda N, Osuga K, Higashihara H, Tomoda K, Mikami K, Nakazawa T, Nakamura H, Tomiyama N. Transarterial chemoembolization with cisplatin as second-line treatment for hepatocellular carci-noma unresponsive to chemoembolization with epirubicin-Lipiodol emulsion. Cardiovasc Intervent Radiol. 2012;35:82–9.
27. Doyon D, Mouzon A, Jourde AM, Regensberg C, Frileux C. Hepatic, arterial embolization in patients with malignant liver tumours (author's transl). Ann Radiol (Paris). 1974;17:593–603.
28. Nakakuma K, Tashiro S, Hiraoka T, Uemura K, Konno T, Miyauchi Y, et al. Studies on anticancer treatment with an oily anticancer drug injected into the ligated feeding hepatic artery for liver cancer. Cancer. 1983;52:2193–200.
29. Kan Z, Sato M, Ivancev K, Uchida B, Hedgpeth P, Lunderquist A, et al. Distribution and effect of iodized poppyseed oil in the liver after hepatic artery embolization: experimental study in several animal species. Radiology. 1993;186:861–6.
30. Kan Z, McCuskey PA, Wright KC, Wallace S. Role of Kupffer cells in iodized oil embolization. Investig Radiol. 1994;29:990–3.
31. Ohishi H, Uchida H, Yoshimura H, Ohue S, Ueda J, Katsuragi M, et al. Hepatocellular carcinoma detected by iodized oil. Use of anticancer agents. Radiology. 1985;154:25–9.
32. De Baere T, Zhang X. Quantification of tumor uptake of iodized oils and emulsions of iodized oils: experimental study. Radiology. 1996;201:731–5.
33. Terayama N, Matsui O, Gabata T, Kobayashi S, Sanada J, Ueda K, Kadoya M, Kawamori Y. Accumulation of iodized oil within the nonneo-plastic liver adjacent to hepatocellular carcinoma via the drainage routes of the tumor after transcatheter arterial embolization. Cardiovasc Intervent Radiol. 2001;24:383–7.
34. Miyayama S, Matsui O, Yamashiro M, Ryu Y, Kaito K, Ozaki K, Takeda T, Yoneda N, Notsumata K, Toya D, et al. Ultraselective transcatheter arterial chemoembolization with a 2-F tip microcatheter for small hepatocellular carcinomas: relationship between local tumor recurrence and visualization of the portal vein with iodized oil. J Vasc Interv Radiol. 2007;18:365–76.
35. Yoshida K. Isolated arteries originating from the intrahepatic arteries: anatomy, function, and importance in intervention. J Vasc Interv Radiol 2018; Miyayama S, Matsui O. Superselective conventional transarterial chemoemboliza-tion for hepatocellular carcinoma: Rationale, technique, and outcome. J Vasc Interv Radiol. 2016;27:1269–1278.
36. Miyayama S, Yamashiro M, Okuda M, Abrano H, Shigenari N, Morinaga K, Matsui O. Anastomosis between the hepatic artery and the extrahepatic col-lateral or between extrahepatic collaterals: obser-vation on angiography. J Med Imag Radiat Oncol. 2009;53:271–82.

37. De Baere T, Arai Y. Treatment of liver tumors with Lipiodol TACE: technical recommendations from experts opinion. Cardiovasc Intervent Radiol. 2016;239:334–43.
38. Demachi H, Matsui O, Abo H, Tatsu H. Simulation model based on non-Newtonian fluid mechanics applied to the evaluation of the embolic effect of emulsions of iodized oil and anticancer drug. Cardiovasc Intervent Radiol. 2000;23:285–90.
39. Minamiguchi K, Tanaka T, Nishiofuku H, Fukuoka Y, Taiji R, Matsumoto T, Saito N, Taguchi H, Marugami N, Hirai T, Kichikawa K. Comparison of embolic effect between water-in-oil emulsion and microspheres in transarterial embolization for rat hepatocellular carcinoma model. Hepatol Res. 2020 Nov;50(11):1297–305.
40. de Baere T, Dufaux J, Roche A, Counnord JL, Berthault MF, Denys A, Pappas P. Circulatory alterations induced by intra-arterial injection of iodized oil and emulsions of iodized oil and doxorubicin: experimental study. Radiology. 1995 Jan;194(1):165–70.
41. Renzulli M, Peta G, Vasuri F, Marasco G, Caretti D, Bartalena L, Spinelli D, Giampalma E, D'Errico A, Golfieri R. Standardization of conventional chemoembolization for hepatocellular carcinoma. Ann Hepatol. 2021 May-Jun;22:100278.
42. Coldwell DM, Stokes KR, Yakes WF. Embolotherapy: agents, clinical applications, and techniques. Radiographics. 1994;14:623–43.
43. Kim BK, Kim SU, Kim KA, Chung YE, Kim MJ, Park MS, Park JY, Kim DY, Ahn SH, Kim MD, et al. Complete response at first chemoembolization is still the most robust predictor for favorable outcome in hepatocellular carcinoma. J Hepatol. 2015;62:1304–10.
44. Kojiro M, Sugihara S, Kakizoe S, Nakashima O, Kiyomatsu K. Hepatocellular carcinoma with sarcomatous change: a special reference to the relationship with anticancer therapy. Cancer Chemother Pharmacol. 1989;23(Suppl):S4–8.
45. Zen C, Zen Y, Mitry RR, Corbeil D, Karbanová J, O'Gray J, Karani J, Kane P, Heaton N, Portmann BC, et al. Mixed phenotype hepatocellular carcinoma after transarterial chemoembolization and liver transplantation. Liver Transpl. 2011;17:943–54.
46. Sergio A, Cristofori C, Cardin R, Pivetta G, Ragazzi R, Baldan A, Girardi L, Cillio U, Burra P, Giacomin A, et al. Transcatheter arterial chemoembolization (TACE) in hepatocellular carcinoma (HCC): the role of angiogenesis and invasiveness. Am J Gastroenterol. 2008;103:914–21.
47. Wang B, Xu H, Gao ZQ, Ning HF, Sun YQ, Cao GW. Increased expression of vascular endothelial growth factor in hepatocellular carcinoma after transcatheter arterial chemoembolization. Acta Radiol. 2008;49:523–9.
48. Miyayama S. Ultraselective conventional transarterial chemoembolization: when and how? Clin Mol Hepatol. 2019;25:344–53.
49. Takeuchi Y, Arai Y, Inaba Y, Ohno K, Maeda T, Itai Y. Extrahepatic arterial supply to the liver: observation with a unified CT and angiography system during temporary balloon occlusion of the proper hepatic artery. Radiology. 1998;209:121–8.
50. Yamakado K, Miyayama S, Hirota S, Mizunuma K, Nakamura K, Inaba Y, Maeda H, Matsuo K, Nishida N, Aramaki T, et al. Hepatic arterial embolization for unresectable hepatocellular carcinomas: Do technical factors affect prognosis? Jpn J Radiol. 2012;30:560–6.
51. Miyayama S, Yamashiro M, Okuda M, Yoshie Y, Sugimori N, Igarashi S, Nakashima Y, Notsumata K, Toya D, Tanaka N, et al. Chemoembolization for the treatment of large hepatocellular carcinoma. J Vasc Interv Radiol. 2010;21:1226–34.
52. Hidaka T, Anai H, Sakaguchi H, Sueyoshi S, Tanaka T, Yamamoto K, Morimoto K, Nishiofuku H, Maeda S, Nagata T, et al. Efficacy of combined bland embolization and chemoembolization for huge (10 cm) hepatocellular carcinoma. Minim Invasive Ther Allied Technol. 2020;30:221.
53. Shaib Y, El-Serag HB. The epidemiology of cholangiocarcinoma. Semin Liver Dis 2004;24:115–125; Bridgewater J, Galle PR, Khan SA, et al.: Guidelines for the diagnosis and management of intrahepatic cholangiocarcinoma. J Hepatol. 2014;60:1268–89.
54. Currie BM, Soulen MC. Decision Making: Intra-arterial Therapies for Cholangiocarcinoma—TACE and TARE. Semin Intervent Radiol. 2017;34:92–100.
55. Grobmyer SR, Wang L, Gonen M, et al. Perihepatic lymph node assessment in patients undergoing partial hepatectomy for malignancy. Ann Surg. 2006;244(02):260–4.
56. Razumilava N, Gores GJ. Cholangiocarcinoma. Lancet. 2014;383(9935):2168–79.
57. Hyder O, Marsh JW, Salem R, et al. Intra-arterial therapy for advanced intrahepatic cholangiocarcinoma: a multi- institutional analysis. Ann Surg Oncol. 2013;20:3779–86.
58. Gusani NJ, Balaa FK, Steel JL, et al. Treatment of unresectable cholangiocarcinoma with gemcitabine- based transcatheter arterial chemoembolization (TACE): a single-institution experience. J Gastrointest Surg. 2008;12:129–37.
59. Herber S, Otto G, Schneider J, et al. Transarterial chemoembolization (TACE) for inoperable intrahepatic cholangiocarcinoma. Cardiovasc Intervent Radiol. 2007;30:1156–65.
60. Scheuermann U, Kaths JM, Heise M, et al. Comparison of resection and transarterial chemoembolisation in the treatment of advanced intrahepatic cholangiocarcinoma–a single-center experience. Eur J Surg Oncol. 2013;39:593–600.
61. Park SY, Kim JH, Yoon HJ, et al. Transarterial chemoembolization versus supportive therapy in the palliative treatment of unresectable intrahepatic cholangiocarcinoma. Clin Radiol. 2011;66:322–8.
62. Shen WF, Zhong W, Liu Q, et al. Adjuvant transcatheter arterial chemoembolization for intrahepatic chol-

angiocarcinoma after curative surgery: retrospective control study. World J Surg. 2011;35:2083–91.
63. Yang GW, Zhao Q, Qian S, et al. Percutaneous microwave ablation combined with simultaneous transarterial chemoembolization for the treatment of advanced intrahepatic cholangiocarcinoma. Onco Targets Ther. 2015;8:1245–50.
64. Vogl TJ, Naguib NN, Nour-Eldin NE, et al. Transarterial chemoembolization in the treatment of patients with unresectable cholangiocarcinoma: results and prognostic factors governing treatment success. Int J Cancer. 2012;131:733–40.
65. Burger I, Hong K, Schulick R, et al. Transcatheter arterial chemoembolization in unresectable cholangiocarcinoma: initial experience in a single institution. J Vasc Interv Radiol. 2005;16:353–61.
66. Kiefer MV, Albert M, McNally M, et al. Chemoembolization of intrahepatic cholangiocarcinoma with cisplatinum, doxorubicin, mitomycin C, ethiodol, and polyvinyl alcohol: a 2-center study. Cancer. 2011;117:1498–505.
67. Seidensticker R, Seidensticker M, Doegen K, et al. Extensive use of interventional therapies improves survival in Unresectable or recurrent intrahepatic cholangiocarcinoma. Gastroenterol Res Pract. 2016;2016:8732521.
68. Kloeckner R, Ruckes C, Kronfeld K, et al. Selective internal radiotherapy (SIRT) versus transarterial chemoembolization (TACE) for the treatment of intrahepatic cholangiocellular carcinoma (CCC): study protocol for a randomized controlled trial. Trials. 2014;15:311.
69. Khan SA, Thomas HC, Davidson BR, et al. Cholangiocarcinoma. Lancet. 2005;366:1303–14.
70. Dingle BH, Rumble RB, Brouwers MC. The role of gemcitabine in the treatment of cholangiocarcinoma and gallbladder cancer: a systematic review. Can J Gastroenterol. 2005;19:711–6.
71. Bray F, Ferlay J, Soerjomataram I, Siegel RL, Torre LA, Jemal A. Global cancer statistics 2018: GLOBOCAN estimates of incidence and mortality worldwide for 36 cancers in 185 countries. CA Cancer J Clin. 2018 Nov;68(6):394–424.
72. Ferlay J, Soerjomataram I, Dikshit R, et al. Cancer incidence and mortality worldwide: sources, methods and major patterns in GLOBOCAN 2012. Int J Cancer. 2015;136:359–86.
73. Torre LA, Bray F, Siegel RL, Ferlay J, Lortet-Tieulent J, Jemal A. Global cancer statistics, 2012. CA Cancer J Clin. 2015;65:87–108.
74. Printz C. National comprehensive cancer network guidelines for small intestine cancers reflect new findings. Cancer. 2020;126:241.
75. Engstrand J, Nilsson H, Stromberg C, et al. Colorectal cancer liver metastases–a population-based study on incidence, management and survival. BMC Canc. 2018;18:78.
76. Misiakos EP, Karidis NP, Kouraklis G. Current treatment for colorectal liver metastases. World J Gastroenterol. 2011;17:4067–75.
77. Alsina J, Choti MA. Liver-directed therapies in colorectal cancer. Semin Oncol. 2011;38:561–7.
78. Vogl TJ, Gruber T, Balzer JO, Eichler K, Hammerstingl R, Zangos S. Repeated transarterial chemoembolization in the treatment of liver metastases of colorectal cancer: prospective study. Radiology. 2009;250:281–9.
79. Sanz-Altamira PM, Spence LD, Huberman MS, et al. Selective chemoembolization in the management of hepatic metastases in refractory colorectal carcinoma: a phase II trial. Dis Colon Rectum. 1997;40:770–5.
80. Tellez C, Benson AB 3rd, Lyster MT, et al. Phase II trial of chemoembolization for the treatment of metastatic colorectal carcinoma to the liver and review of the literature. Cancer. 1998;82:1250–9.
81. Albert M, Kiefer MV, Sun W, et al. Chemoembolization of colorectal liver metastases with cisplatin, doxorubicin, mitomycin C, ethiodol, and polyvinyl alcohol. Cancer. 2011;117:343–52.
82. van Hazel GA, Heinemann V, Sharma NK, et al. SIRFLOX. J Clin Oncol. 2016;34:1723e1731.
83. Wasan HS, Gibbs P, Sharma NK, et al. First-line selective internal radiotherapy plus chemotherapy versus chemotherapy alone in patients with liver metastases from colorectal cancer (FOXFIRE, SIRFLOX, FOXFIRE-Global). Lancet Oncol. 2017;18:1159e1171.
84. Sullivan RD, Norcross JW, Watkins E. Chemotherapy of metastatic liver cancer by prolonged hepatic-artery infusion. N Engl J Med. 1964;270:321e327.
85. Kemeny NE, Niedzwiecki D, Hollis DR, et al. Hepatic arterial infusion versus systemic therapy for hepatic metastases from colorectal cancer: a randomized trial of efficacy, quality of life, and molecular markers (CALGB 9481). J Clin Oncol. 2006;24:1395e1403.
86. Levi FA, Boige V, Hebbar M, et al. Conversion to resection of liver metastases from colorectal cancer with hepatic artery infusion of combined chemotherapy and systemic cetuximab in multicenter trial OPTILIV. Ann Oncol. 2016;27:267e274.
87. Levy J, Zuckerman J, Garfinkle R, Acuna SA, Touchette J, Vanounou T, Pelletier SS. Intra-arterial therapies for unresectable and chemorefractory colorectal cancer liver metastases: a systematic review and meta-analysis. HPB. 2018;20:905–15.
88. Bavisotto L, Patel N, Althaus S, Coldwell DM, Nghiem HV, Thompson T, Storer B, Thomas CR Jr. Hepatic transcatheter arterial chemoembolization alternating with systemic protracted continuous infusion 5-fluorouracil for gastrointestinal malignancies metastatic to liver: a phase II trial of the Puget Sound oncology consortium (PSOC 1104). Clin Cancer Res. 1999;5(1):95–109.
89. Hunt T, Flowerdew A, Birch S, Williams J, Mullee M, Taylor I. Prospective randomized controlled trial of hepatic arterial embolization or infusion chemotherapy with 5-fluorouracil and degradable starch

microspheres for colorectal liver metastases. Br J Surg. 1990;77(7):779–82.
90. Hong K, McBride J, Georgiades C, Reyes DK, Herman JM, Kamel IR, Geschwind JF. Salvage therapy for liver-dominant colorectal metastatic adenocarcinoma: comparison between trans-catheter arterial chemoembolization *versus* yttrium-90 radioembolization. J Vasc Interv Radiol. 2009;20(3):360–7.
91. Nishiofuku H, Tanaka T, Matsuoka M, Otsuji T, Anai H, Sueyoshi S, Inaba Y, Koyama F, Sho M, Nakajima Y, Kichikawa K. Transcatheter arterial chemo-embolization using cisplatin powder mixed with degradable starch microspheres for colorectal liver metastases after FOLFOX failure: results of a phase I/II study. J Vasc Interv Radiol. 2013;24(1):56–65.
92. Salman HS, Cynamon J, Jagust M, Bakal C, Rozenblit A, Kaleya R, Negassa A, Wadler S. Randomized phase II trial of embolization therapy *versus* chemo-embolization therapy in previously treated patients with colorectal carcinoma metastatic to the liver. Clin Colorectal Cancer. 2002;2(3):173–9.
93. NCCN Clinical Practice Guidelines in Oncology (NCCN Guidelines). Neuroendocrine Tumors, Version 2. 2016. Available at: https://www. nccn.org/professionals/physician_gls/pdf/neuroendocrine.pdf. Accessed June 25, 2017.
94. Kennedy A, Bester L, Salem R, et al. Role of hepatic intra-arterial therapies in metastatic neuroendocrine tumours (NET): guidelines from the NET-liver-metastases consensus conference. HPB (Oxford). 2015;17:29–37.
95. Patel K, Sullivan K, Berd D, et al. Chemoembolization of the hepatic artery with BCNU for metastatic uveal melanoma: results of a phase II study. Melanoma Res. 2005;15:297–304.
96. Gonsalves CF, Eschelman DJ, Thornburg B, Frangos A, Sato T. Uveal melanoma metastatic to the liver: chemoembolization with 1,3-bis- (2-chloroethyl)-1-nitrosourea. AJR Am J Roentgenol. 2015;205:429–33.
97. Sharma KV, Gould JE, Harbour JW, et al. Hepatic arterial chemo- embolization for management of metastatic melanoma. AJR Am J Roentgenol. 2008;190:99–104.
98. Gupta S, Bedikian AY, Ahrar J, et al. Hepatic artery chemoembolization in patients with ocular melanoma metastatic to the liver: response, survival, and prognostic factors. Am J Clin Oncol. 2010;33:474–80.
99. Sato T. Locoregional management of hepatic metastasis from primary uveal melanoma. Semin Oncol. 2010;37:127–38.
100. Agarwala SS, Eggermont AM, O'Day S, Zager JS. Metastatic melanoma to the liver: a contemporary and comprehensive review of surgical, systemic, and regional therapeutic options. Cancer. 2014;120:781–9.

7 Drug-Eluting Embolic TACE (DEB-TACE)

Marta Burrel and Patricia Bermúdez

7.1 TACE with Drug-Eluting Microspheres (DEM-TACE)

Drug-eluting microspheres were developed in the early 2000 to overcome the limitations of conventional TACE, such as lack of standardization of the technique and nonsimultaneous administration of the chemotherapeutic and embolic agents. Since objective response had been reported as an independent factor for survival [1], the aim of technical refinement was to selectively deliver drug into the tumor, thus achieving better response, avoiding its systemic toxicity.

Drug-eluting microspheres are embolic agents composed of a hydrophilic, ionic polymer that can bind anthracyclines via an ion exchange mechanism, thanks to the interaction of the cationic drug with the anionic functional groups of the microspheres. The interaction is reversible in ion-rich environments such as tumors, where the drug is slowly released [2].

Currently, various types of drug-eluting embolic agents are commercially available for use with doxorubicin, including DC Bead (BTG, Farnham, UK), HepaSphere (Merit Medical, South Jordan, Utah), LifePearl (Terumo European Interventional Systems, Leuven, Belgium), and Tandem (Boston Scientific, Marlborough, Massachusetts) microspheres, with some differences among them in elution and suspension characteristics [3]. Phase I–II trials evaluating pharmacokinetics, safety, and efficacy have been performed with DC Bead [4, 5] and LifePearl [6].

A more recently developed drug-eluting technology bead is DC Bead LUMI™ (Biocompatibles UK Ltd., UK) that incorporates iodine into its chemical structure, ensuring that is permanently radiopaque. These particles have shown intra- and post-procedural benefits derived from their improved visualization, such as identification of nontarget embolization and identification of undertreated regions that allow real-time modification of the procedure and indication of embolized vessels for subsequent treatments like additional embolization or combination with ablation therapies. They have shown, in small case series, safety and response rates comparable to those published for non-radiopaque beads [7]. A drawback is the limitation of CT evaluation after treatment, given its permanent radiopacity, that may prevent to detect contrast uptake in the tumor [8].

M. Burrel (✉) · P. Bermúdez
Barcelona Liver Cancer Group (BCLC),
Vascular Radiology Unit, Radiology Department,
Hospital Clinic, Barcelona, Spain
e-mail: MBURREL@clinic.cat; pbermude@clinic.cat

P. Lucatelli (ed.), *Transarterial Chemoembolization (TACE)*,
https://doi.org/10.1007/978-3-031-36261-3_7

7.1.1 DEM-TACE in Hepatocellular Carcinoma

7.1.1.1 Drugs

The drug loaded is doxorubicin. While in conventional TACE the dose has to be tailored according to body surface or weight, in DEM-TACE, it is not. In the Precision I study [4], the authors analyzed the concentration of doxorubicin in peripheral blood samples in a group of patients receiving DEM-TACE and others treated with cTACE. The maximum peak concentration was determined 7 min after the start of the drug injection in both groups; the AUC of doxorubicin in peripheral blood was significantly lower in the DEM-TACE group compared to the cTACE, although the dose of drug administered was significantly higher. The two phase I/II trials performing a pharmacokinetic analysis used a conventional dose escalation strategy to evaluate the maximum total dose of doxorubicin and demonstrated the safety of 150 mg as a maximum total dose per session of treatment [4, 5]. This is the current standard applied in clinical practice.

Each vial of DEM (2 ml of beads) should be loaded with 50–75 mg doxorubicin (loading dose 25–37.5 mg doxorubicin/ml of beads). Depending on the tumor burden, one or two vials are prepared for each treatment session.

The rationale for the use of doxorubicin relies on results from a phase II trial that showed some complete responses using this drug [9] and the lack of evidence of few RCTs comparing different drugs. Recently, an in vitro study showed that idarubicin was the most cytotoxic drug among 10 agents tested [10], and this has been the rationale for the development of idarubicin-loaded beads. Recent studies have shown improved response rates and safety [11], and it stands as a promising chemotherapeutic agent for HCC treatment.

7.1.1.2 Bead Size

The recommended bead size for a standard procedure is 100–300 μm, although individual patient and tumor characteristics must be taken into account and larger beads (300–500 microns) can be also used [12].

The choice of 100–300 μm is based on the demonstration that such small particles are delivered inside the tumor. Accumulative evidence has shown that intratumoral vessels are usually smaller than 300 μm [13, 14] or in close proximity to the tumor margin. The study performed by Malagari et al. proved that 100–300 μm DEM are equally safe compared to larger particles [15]. Of note, in this study, transient elevations of liver enzymes have been reported to be higher with smaller beads, as well as a trend to higher bilirubin levels (p = 0.03–0.04) [15], although these laboratory findings have not proved to impact on survival.

Beads <100 μm permit deeper and more homogeneous vessel penetration with improved drug coverage. However, several studies have shown that patients with neuroendocrine metastases and non-cirrhotic liver [16, 17] treated with small beads develop more complications; this has also been described with Gelfoam powder [18]. Additionally, asymptomatic liver/biliary injuries have been observed in up to 29% of cases [19]. While some authors have shown good tumor response rates and favorable safety and tolerability using 70–150 μm [20–22], others have reported more clinical hepatobiliary complications compared to larger size [23]. A combined embolization approach using 100 μm ± 25 microspheres and followed by 200 μm ± 50 microspheres has been successfully tested; the rationale is that smaller beads would deposit intratumorally increasing the cytotoxic effect, and the larger would occlude the peritumoral arterioles, thus enhancing ischemia [24]. Taking all these considerations together, the choice of <100 μm may be safe in selected cases [19].

7.1.1.3 Procedural Specifications

The evaluation on tumor burden allows for planning the dose as well as the bead size. Since the preparation of DEM is done in a pharmacy hospital and at least 8 h are needed to achieve complete loading of doxorubicin, it is recommended to previously assess the tumor burden on CT/MR examinations in order to choose the bead size and the dose (prepare one or two vials). For this purpose and as a general rule, the aim of the treatment session is to treat all tumors, even if they involve both lobes, and to achieve stasis of the feeders. Nevertheless, we must keep in mind that this treatment endpoint is applicable in patients with preserved hepatic function, which means Child A patients without hepatic decompensation. Therefore, in patients with more advanced liver disease, the treatment endpoint or the indication of treatment by TACE has to be balanced with the hepatic function.

No antibiotic prophylaxis [25, 26] or anti-inflammatory drugs are mandatory prior to treatment. Antibiotic prophylaxis can be considered for patients with past history of biliodigestive derivation, cholecystectomy, sphincterotomy, and HIV. Pain management during the procedure should be individualized for each patient.

Once the angiographic 4- or 5-F catheter is placed in the main hepatic artery, superselective catheterization of the feeders is performed. This should be done using a coaxial microcatheter (2.7–2.4 F). The tip of the microcatheter must be placed as distally as possible (feeding artery, subsegmental, less desirable segmental or lobar level), and this depends on the tumor burden and capacity of navigation through the intrahepatic vessels.

DEM are administered using a 1- to 3-ml syringe, mixed with contrast. Special attention must be taken to specifications according to different companies. In all cases, a good suspension of DEM should be ensured before delivery. Either contrast or saline/water can be added depending on the concentration of beads and fluid density.

The aim during infusion is to deliver the maximum DEM into the target. The infusion must be very slow, with smooth pulses, allowing the normal flow to push the beads into the tumor feeders. Care should be taken to avoid sedimentation of the beads in the syringe by rotating the syringes or using a three-way stopcock to gently suspend the beads in the solution. Beads are administered under continuous fluoroscopic monitoring until stagnation of flow is achieved. At this point, injection must be stopped, regardless of the amount of beads that have been actually administered, to avoid reflux of embolic material [12].

When the treatment is finished, a final angiography has to be performed to assess tumor devascularization. A CBCT without contrast is especially useful for those cases treated with LUMI beads to assess the final deposition of beads. Also, some authors have reported the usefulness of a CBCT immediately at the end of the procedure to assess the bead retention within the tumor [27].

7.1.1.4 Results

The first clinical study reporting the efficacy of DEB-TACE was the Precision I [4], a phase II study; the pharmacokinetic analysis was clearly favorable with the demonstration of doxorubicin maximal concentration in peripheral blood significantly inferior in comparison with cTACE, and the absence of doxorubicin-related systemic side effects. These results were reproduced by Poon et al. [5]. Furthermore, encouraging tumor response rates were reported, and during the early 2010, two European cohort studies showed median overall survival figures that exceeded 40 months [28, 29] that nearly doubled those published in the first two RCT comparing TACE with best supportive care, reported as 28,7 months [1] and 18 months [30]. Of notice, it must be considered that these striking results were obtained in different population (BCLC B patients with limited tumor burden and well-preserved hepatic function) compared to those of the previous decade treated with cTACE, when TACE was applied to less optimal population (more advanced disease and worse liver function), because no other treatment options except best supportive care could be offered. In fact, at the time of the development and application of DEM-TACE, sorafenib was already available as a treatment option for patient refractory to TACE therapy.

During the most recent years, various studies have been performed to compare DEM-TACE with cTACE. Concerning safety profile and tolerance, the results of the Precision V study clearly favored DEM-TACE, reporting significant decrease in serious liver-related adverse events ($P < 0.001$) and systemic side effects ($P = 0.0001$) [31]. The improved tolerance profile of DEM-

TACE has been reproduced in the RCT performed by the Precision Italia Study Group, where the post-procedural pain was more frequent and severe after cTACE [32].

Regarding survival, RCTs have failed to show differences between both modalities of treatment [31–33]. There is a single center retrospective study from Korea including 129 patients that compared both treatment modalities; the authors reported a mean overall survival of 32 months for patients treated with DEM-TACE, and a significantly higher OS in the DEM group than in the cTACE group ($p = 0.005$). The study also reports a high overall response rate using DEM (71% OR, 55% complete and 26% partial response), which was significantly higher in the DEM group than that in the cTACE group ($p < 0.001$), particularly in the intermediate stage [34]. However, the more recent meta-analysis of 12 studies including 8 RCTs has also failed to show differences between both modalities, only highlighting a decreasing trend in favor of DEM-TACE [35].

7.1.1.5 Bland Embolization Versus TACE and Treatment Endpoint

According to published results and guidelines, median survival of BCLC B patients receiving TACE should be not less than 2.5 years [36]. Furthermore, systemic therapies are rapidly developing with high expectations for rapid broadening of the therapeutic armamentarium beyond tyrosine-kinase inhibitors. Currently, ongoing trials are competing with transarterial therapies, and indications for TACE are likely going to be narrowed in the next future (paucinodular HCCs in patients with well-preserved liver function). Finally, it is reported that a complete response after the initial TACE is the most robust predictor of long-term survival [37]. Hence, there is a growing necessity to achieve "curative" results following TACE and to discuss about the treatment endpoint of TACE.

The rationale for the treatment is based on the synergetic effect of the chemotherapeutic (cytotoxic) and embolic (hypoxic-ischemic) agents. However, the usefulness of drug injection is still a matter of debate, and robust data in favor of TACE over bland embolization is still lacking [38, 39].

An RCT conducted in early 2000s comparing TACE, TAE, and BSC was stopped at an interim analysis when clear superiority of TACE over BSC was observed, preventing the comparison between TACE and TAE; only a trend favoring TACE could be observed [1]. Additionally, positive signs of TACE over bland embolization have been reported. A prospective trial that randomized patients either to DEB-TACE or bland embolization showed a significant lower recurrence rate and longer time to progression for patients treated with DEB-TACE [40]. A study that analyzed retrospectively a cohort of transplanted patients that had been treated with either TACE or bland embolization reported higher tumor necrosis and improved recurrence-free survival after liver transplant when DEB-TACE was the treatment applied [41]. Hence, the standard of care in the majority of centers is still TACE over bland embolization.

Vascular endothelial growth factor (VEGF) is an important mediator of tumor angiogenesis [42]. A prospective study to evaluate the prognostic significance of pretreatment serum VEGF levels in patients with HCC treated with TACE reported that high levels of VEGF were associated to worse survival. On the other hand, it has been reported that there is an increased expression of VEGF in residual viable tumor after TACE [43]. Therefore, incomplete tumor devascularization could potentially stimulate tumor proliferation in the residual viable tissue. This could also happen when treatment is scheduled in two sessions to treat each lobe separately, in such cases tumor proliferation in the initially untreated lobes.

Based on all these considerations, the endpoint of the treatment should be to achieve complete tumor devascularization together with the injection of the maximum amount of the chemotherapeutic agent. If the stasis endpoint is not obtained after injection of the scheduled volume of loaded beads, additional unloaded beads would be injected until the embolization endpoint has been reached. Even so, and because there is not definite evidence, some groups still recommend to schedule the patient for a repeat course of treatment once the total amount of drug is injected.

7.1.2 DEM-TACE in Other Tumors

7.1.2.1 DEM-TACE for Intrahepatic Cholangiocarcinoma

Clinical indications for transarterial chemoembolization or embolization of ICC include surgically unresectable or inoperable liver tumors with liver-dominant disease. An important consideration in patients with ICC is the presence of biliary obstruction, which is a contraindication for TACE due to the risk of abscess or infectious disease. In patients with repaired biliary obstruction, periprocedural intravenous antibiotic therapy may lower the risk of complications [44].

The most widely and preferred drug is, again, doxorubicin. Other drugs that have been tested with good results are oxaliplatin and epirubicin.

Evidence of the efficacy of DEM-TACE is based on small series reporting a median survival of 11–13 months that appears to increase when combining systemic chemotherapy, although toxicity increases when combined therapy is applied. The series published are small and the drug loaded differs among them, preventing an adequate interpretation of the results [45].

However, the outcomes of different intra-arterial modalities for the treatment of ICC still need to be standardized and compared, and indications have to be defined. A meta-analysis comparing different intra-arterial therapies for ICC showed a trend favoring HAI (hepatic artery infusion) over DEM-TACE [46].

DEM-TACE for Colorectal Cancer Liver Metastases

Irinotecan-loaded drug-eluting bead (DEBIRI) embolization was developed to treat colorectal metastases to the liver. The mechanism of action is based on the effect of irinotecan, which is activated by normal liver parenchyma via hydrolysis.

The technical aspects of DEBIRI are still under discussion. The recommended irinotecan dose delivery is 100 mg [46], but no dose escalation studies have been performed so far. Concerning dose of irinotecan and size of beads, and according to results of a prospective registry, small beads (75–150 or 100–300 micron) that allow for increased dose delivery are recommended [48]. The general recommendation is to perform nonselective embolization for normal hepatocytes to activate the drug, and to cover lesions not detected at imaging, although this has not been conclusively proven. Finally, the most recommended treatment regimen provides two treatment sessions for each lobe (in case of bilobar disease, a total of four treatments are scheduled, where alternated lobes are treated every 2 weeks) [47].

Although the initial DEBIRI published data were promising, the heterogeneity of study designs and results hinder the consensus on the treatment. A prospective randomized study comparing DEBIRI with FOLFIRI in patients that had received previous systemic chemotherapy without irinotecan and had liver-only metastatic disease showed significant PFS and OS of the liver-directed therapy [49]. However, these results were not reproduced and treatment is currently applied in a salvage setting. Another matter of debate is whether the therapy has to be applied in liver-only or liver-dominant disease [50].

DEM-TACE for Neuroendocrine Tumor Liver Metastases

Indications for intra-arterial therapy in patients with liver metastases from NET include those with progressive disease or symptoms refractory to medical treatment. DEM-TACE is one of the approaches proposed and applied in many institutions due to its excellent pharmacokinetic profile; however, a study published in 2017 that compared DEB-TACE with cTACE showed more benefit of the latter modality [51]. Although there is no definite data to recommend TACE over TARE for the treatment of liver metastases from NET, the most recent meta-analysis of six trials has shown a significant survival benefit and less adverse effects of TACE in comparison to TARE [52].

Prophylactic use of somatostatin analogues 24–48 h before TACE is recommended in patients with functional tumors, to avoid an acute carcinoid crisis triggered by the procedure. It is also mandatory to perform screening and treatment for carcinoid heart disease [53]. Of note, the concomitant treatment of somatostatin analogues has shown a prolonged time to liver progression in patients receiving TACE [54].

The factor that limits the application of DEM-TACE for this type of tumors is the increased risk of ischemic biliary injury. This is related to the occlusion of peribiliary plexus that is not enlarged in patients with normal (non-cirrhotic) liver parenchyma; conversely, in cirrhosis, the hypertrophied peribiliary plexus protects against the ischemic injury. Liver/biliary injuries have been reported as independently associated with DEB-TACE and NETs [55]. It has been described in the literature the increased risk of hepatobiliary events in comparing patients with cirrhotic liver and HCC, even using the same bead size and endpoint. This is the rationale for a proposed different technical endpoint of DEM-TACE in this type of tumors (i.e., drug delivery instead of vascular stasis): accordingly, fewer adverse events have been reported when free-flow arterial circulation has been achieved after TACE instead of vascular stasis [56].

References

1. Llovet JM, Real MI, Montana X, Planas R, Coll S, Aponte J, et al. Arterial embolisation or chemoembolisation versus symptomatic treatment in patients with unresectable hepatocellular carcinoma: a randomised controlled trial. Lancet. 2002;359:1734–9.
2. Lewis AL, Gonzalez MV, Lloyd AW, Hall B, Tang Y, Willis SL, et al. DC bead: in vitro characterization of a drug-delivery device for transarterial chemoembolization. J Vasc Interv Radiol. 2006;17:335–42.
3. DeBaere T, Plotkin S, Yu R, Sutter A, Wu Y, Cruise G. An in vitro evaluation of four types of drug-eluting microspheres loaded with doxorubicin. J Vasc Interv Radiol. 2016;27:1425–31.
4. Varela M, Real MI, Burrel M, Forner A, Sala M, Brunet M, et al. Chemoembolization of hepatocellular carcinoma with drug eluting beads: efficacy and doxorubicin pharmacokinetics. J Hepatol. 2007;46:474–81.
5. Poon RT, Tso WK, Pang RW, et al. A phase I/II trial of chemoembolisation for hepatocellular carcinoma using a novel intra-arterial drug-eluting bead. Clin Gastroenterol Hepatol. 2007;5:1100–8.
6. Malagari K, Burrel M, Reig M, Brunet M, Denys A, Bruix J. LIFEPEARL-DOXO STUDY pharmacokinetic study of doxorubicin in the treatment of unresectable HCC by LifePearl® interim analyses. Presented at CIRSE annual meeting, Lisbon, 22-25 Sept 2018.
7. Reicher J, Mafeld S, Priona G, Reeves HL, Manas DM, Jackson R, Littler P. Early experience of trans-arterial chemo-embolisation for hepatocellular carcinoma with a novel radiopaque bead. Cardiovasc Intervent Radiol. 2019;42:1563–70.
8. Moschouris H, Malagari K, Dimakis A, et al. Transarterial chemoembolization of hcc with radiopaque microspheres: evaluation with computed tomography and the complementary role of contrast-enhanced ultrasonography. Cardiovasc Intervent Radiol. 43(7):1075–83.
9. Olweny CL, Toya T, Katongole-Mbidde E, Mugerwa J, Kyalwazi SK, Cohen H. Treatment of hepatocellular carcinoma with Adriamycin: preliminary communication. Cancer. 1975;36(4):1250–7.
10. Boulin M, Guiu S, Chauffert B, et al. Screening of anticancer drugs for chemoembolization of hepatocellular carcinoma. Anti-Cancer Drugs. 2011;22(8):741–8.
11. Guiu B, Chevallier P, Assenat P, et al. Idarubicin-loaded beads for chemoembolization of hepatocellular carcinoma: the IDASPHERE II single-arm phase II trial. Radiology. 2019;291:801–8.
12. Lencioni R, De Baere T, Burrel M, Caridi J, et al. Transcatheter treatment of hepatocellular carcinoma with doxorubicin-loaded DC bead (DEBDOX): technical recommendations. Cardiovasc Intervent Radiol. 2012;35:980–5.
13. Lee KH, Liapi E, Ventura VP, et al. Evaluation of different calibrated spherical polyvinyl alcohol microspheres in transcatheter arterial chemoembolization: VX2 tumor model in rabbit liver. J Vasc Interv Radiol. 2008;19(7):1065–9.
14. Lee KH, Liapi E, Vossen JA, et al. Distribution of iron oxide-containing Embosphere particles after transcatheter arterial embolization in an animal model of liver cancer: evaluation with MR imaging and implication for therapy. J Vasc Interv Radiol. 2008;19(10):1490–6.
15. Malagari, et al. Safety profile of sequential transcatheter chemoembolization with DC bead: results of 237 hepatocellular carcinoma (HCC) patients. Cardiovasc Intervent Radiol. 2010;34:774.
16. Bhagat, et al. Phase II study of chemoembolization with drug-eluting beads in patients with hepatic neuroendocrine metastases: high incidence of biliary injury. Cardiovasc Intervent Radiol. 2013 Apr;36(2):449–59.
17. Sakamoto I, et al. Intrahepatic Biloma formation (bile duct necrosis) after transcatheter arterial chemoembolization. AJR Am J Roentgenol. 2003;181(1):79–87.

18. Makuuchi M, Sukigara M, Mori T, et al. Bile duct necrosis: complication of transcatheter hepatic arterial embolization. Radiology. 1985;56(2):331–4.
19. Odisio BV, Ashton A, Yan Y, et al. Transarterial hepatic chemoembolization with 70-150 μm drug-eluting beads: assessment of clinical safety and liver toxicity profile. J Vasc Interv Radiol. 2015 Jul;26(7):965–71.
20. Aliberti C, Carandina R, Lonardi S et al. Transarterial chemoembolization with small drug-eluting beads in patients with hepatocellular carcinoma: experience from a cohort of 421 patients at an Italian center.
21. Spreafico C, Cascella T, Facciorusso A, et al. Transarterial chemoembolization for hepatocellular carcinoma with a new generation of beads: clinical–radiological outcomes and safety profile. Cardiovasc Intervent Radiol. 2015;38:129–34.
22. Urbano J, Echevarria-Uraga J, Ciampi-Dopazo JJ. Multicentre prospective study of drug-eluting bead chemoembolisation safety using tightly calibrated small microspheres in non-resectable hepatocellular carcinoma. Eur J Radiol. 2020;126:108966.
23. Deipolyi A, Oklu R, Al-Ansari S, et al. Safety and efficacy of 70-150 μm and 100-300 μm drug-eluting bead Transarterial chemoembolization for hepatocellular carcinoma. JVIR. 2015 Apr;26(4):516–22.
24. Lucatelli P, Argirò R, De Rubeis G, et al. Polyethylene glycol Epirubicin-loaded Transcatheter arterial chemoembolization procedures utilizing a combined approach with 100 and 200 μm microspheres: a promising alternative to current standards. J Vasc Interv Radiol. 2019 Mar;30(3):305–13.
25. Shelgikar CS, Loehle J, Scoggins CR, McMasters KM, Martin RC 2nd. Empiric antibiotics for transarterial embolization in hepatocellular carcinoma: indicated? J Surg Res. 2009;151:121–4.
26. Castells A, Bruix J, Ayuso C, Bru C, Montanya X, Boix L, et al. Transarterial embolization for hepatocellular carcinoma. Antibiotic prophylaxis and clinical meaning of postembolization fever. J Hepatol. 1995;22:410–5.
27. Lucatelli P, Corona M, Argirò R, Anzidei M, Vallati G, Fanelli F, Bezzi M, Catalano C. Impact of 3D rotational angiography on liver embolization procedures: review of technique and applications. Cardiovasc Intervent Radiol. 2015 Jun;38(3):523–35.
28. Burrel M, Reig M, Forner A, et al. Survival of patients with hepatocellular carcinoma treated by transarterial chemoembolisation (TACE) using drug eluting beads. Implications for clinical practice and trial design. J Hepatol. 2012;56:1330–5.
29. Malagari K, Pomoni M, Moschouris H, et al. Chemoembolization with doxorubicin-eluting beads for unresectable hepatocellular carcinoma: five-year survival analysis. Cardiovasc Intervent Radiol. 2012;35:1119–28.
30. Lo CM, Ngan H, Tso WK, et al. Randomized controlled trial of transarterial lipiodol chemoembolization for unresectable hepatocellular carcinoma. Hepatology. 2002;35:1164–71.
31. Lammer J, Malagari K, Vogl T, et al. PRECISION V investigators. Prospective randomized study of doxorubicin- eluting-bead embolization in the treatment of hepatocellular carcinoma: results of the PRECISION V study. Cardiovasc Intervent Radiol. 2010;33:41–52.
32. Golfieri R, Giampalma E, Renzulli M, Cioni R, Bargellini I, Bartolozzi C, Breatta AD, Gandini G, Nani R, Gasparini D, Cucchetti A, Bolondi L, Trevisani F, Precision Italia Study Group. Randomised controlled trial of doxorubicin-eluting beads vs conventional chemoembolisation for hepatocellular carcinoma. Br J Cancer. 2014;111:255–64.
33. Sacco R, Bargellini I, Bertini M, et al. Conventional versus doxorubicin-eluting bead transarterial chemoembolization for hepatocellular carcinoma. J Vasc Interv Radiol. 2011;22:1545–52.
34. Song MJ, Chun HJ, Song DS, Kim HY, Yoo SH, Park CH, Bae SH, Choi JY, Chang UI, Yang JM, Lee HG, Yoon SK. Comparative study between doxorubicin-eluting beads and conventional transarterial chemoembolization for treatment of hepatocellular carcinoma. J Hepatol. 2012;57:1244–50.
35. Faciorusso A, Di Maso M, Muscatiello N. Drug-eluting beads versus conventional chemoembolization for the treatment of unresectable hepatocellular carcinoma: a meta-analysis. Dig Liver Dis. 2016;48:571–7.
36. Reig M, Forner A, Rimola A, et al. BCLC strategy for prognosis prediction and treatment recommendation: the 2022 update. J Hepatol. 2022 Mar;76(3):681–93.
37. Kim BK, Kim SU, Kima KA, Chung YE, Kim MJ, Park MS, Park J, Dim DY, Ahn SH, Kim MD, et al. Complete response at first chemoembolization is still the most robust predictor for favorable outcome in hepatocellular carcinoma. J Hepatol. 2015;62:1304–10.
38. Brown KT, Do RK, Gonen M, Covey AM, Getrajdman GI, Sofocleous CT, Jarnagin WR, D'Angelica MI, Allen PJ, Erinjeri JP, Brody LA, O'Neill GP, Johnson KN, Garcia AR, Beattie C, Zhao B, Solomon SB, Schwartz LH, DeMatteo R, Abou- Alfa GK. Randomized trial of hepatic artery embolization for hepatocellular carcinoma using doxorubicin-eluting microspheres compared with embolization with microspheres alone. J Clin Oncol. 2016;34:2046–53.
39. Marelli L, Stigliano R, Triantos C, Senzolo M, Cholongitas E, Davies N, et al. Transarterial therapy for hepatocellular carcinoma: which technique is more effective? A systematic review of cohort and randomized studies. Cardiovasc Intervent Radiol. 2007;30:6–25.
40. Malagari K, Pomoni M, Kelekis A, Pomoni A, Dourakis S, Spyridopoulos T, Moschouris H, Emmanouil E, Rizos S, Kelekis D. Prospective randomized comparison of chemoembolization with doxorubicin-eluting beads and bland embolization with BeadBlock for hepatocellular carcinoma. Cardiovasc Intervent Radiol. 2010;33:541–51.
41. Nicolini A, Martinetti L, Crespi S, Maggioni M, Sangiovanni A. Transarterial chemoembolization with

epirubicin-eluting beads versus transarterial embolization before liver transplantation for hepatocellular carcinoma. J Vasc Interv Radiol. 2010;21:327–32.
42. Poon RT-P, Lau C, Yu W-C, et al. High serum levels of vascular endothelial growth factor predict poor response to transarterial chemoembolization in hepatocellular carcinoma: a prospective study. Oncol Rep. 2004;11:1077–84.
43. Wang B, Xu H, Gao ZQ. Increased expression of vascular endothelial growth factor in hepatocellular carcinoma after transcatheter arterial chemoembolization. Acta Radiol. 2008 Jun;49(5):523–9.
44. Gaba RC, Lokken P, Ryan M, et al. Quality improvement guidelines for Transarterial chemoembolization and embolization of hepatic malignancy. J Vasc Interv Radiol. 2017;28:1210–23.
45. Boehm LM, Jayakrishnan TT, Miura JT, Zacharias AJ, Johnston FM, Turaga KK, Gamlin C. Comparative effectiveness of hepatic artery-based therapies for unresectable intrahepatic cholangiocarcinoma. J Surg Oncol. 2015 Feb;111(2):213–20.
46. Savic LJ, Chapiro J, Geschwind JF. Intra-arterial embolotherapy for intrahepatic cholangiocarcinoma: update and future prospects. Hepatobiliary Surg Nutr. 2017 Feb;6(1):7–21.
47. Lencioni R, Aliberti C, de Baere T, et al. Transarterial treatment of colorectal cancer liver metastases with irinotecan-loaded drug- eluting beads: technical recommendations. J Vasc Interv Radiol. 2014;25(3):365–9.
48. Akinwande OK, Philips P, Duras P, Pluntke S, Scoggins C, Marin RC. Small versus large-sized drug-eluting beads (DEBIRI) for the treatment of hepatic colorectal metastases: a propensity score matching analysis. Cardiovasc Interv Radiol. 2015;38(2):361–71.
49. Fiorentini G, Aliberti C, Tilli M, et al. Intra-arterial infusion of irinotecan-loaded drug-eluting beads (DEBIRI) versus intra- venous therapy (FOLFIRI) for hepatic metastases from colorectal cancer: final results of a phase III study. Anticancer Res. 2012;32(4):1387–95.
50. Pereira P, Iezzi R, Manfredi R. The CIREL cohort: a prospective controlled registry studying the Real-life use of irinotecan-loaded chemoembolisation in colorectal cancer liver metastases: interim analysis. Cardiovasc Intervent Radiol. 2021 Jan;44(1):50–62.
51. Minh DD, Chapiro J, Gorodetski B, et al. Intra-arterial therapy of neuroendocrine tumor liver metastases: comparing conventional TACE, drug-eluting beads TACE and yttrium-90 radioembolisation as treatment options using a propensity score analysis model. Eur Radiol. 2017 Dec;27(12):4995–5005.
52. Ngo L, Elnahla A, Attia A, et al. Chemoembolization versus radioembolization for neuroendocrine liver metastases: a meta-analysis comparing clinical outcomes. Ann Surg Oncol. 2021;28:1950–8.
53. de Baere T, Deschamps F, Tselikas L, et al. GEP-NETS update: interventional radiology: role in the treatment of liver metastases from GEP-NETs. Eur J Endocrinol. 2015;172(4):R151–66.
54. Touloupas C, Matthieu F, Hadoux J. Long term efficacy and assessment of tumor response of Transarterial chemoembolization in neuroendocrine liver metastases: a 15-year monocentric experience. Cancers (Basel). 2021;13(21):5366.
55. Guiu B, Deschamps F, Aho S, et al. Liver/biliary injuries following chemoembolisation of endocrine tumours and hepatocellular carcinoma: lipiodol vs. drug-eluting beads. J Hepatol. 2012 Mar;56(3):609–17.
56. Bagdonavicius MJ, Kohan AA, Peralta O, et al. Adverse events and treatment response using different embolization endpoints in a cohort of patients with neuroendocrine liver metastasis treated with drug eluting beads. Abstract Only. 25(3):S1–S268. SIR 2014 Annual Scientific Meeting Program. 22 March 2014–27 March 2014

8 Transarterial Chemoembolization with Degradable Starch Microspheres (DSM-TACE)

Timo Alexander Auer and Federico Collettini

8.1 Introduction

Since its introduction more than 30 years ago, transarterial chemoembolization (TACE) has become a widely accepted locoregional therapy for the palliative treatment of liver cancer. TACE can be performed with a variety of embolic and chemotherapeutic agents, and despite widespread clinical use, there is an ongoing debate about different TACE protocols and how best to deliver the therapy. Currently, two TACE techniques are mainly used in clinical routine: conventional TACE (cTACE) and drug-eluting bead TACE (DEB-TACE). In cTACE, the chemotherapeutic drug is administered intra-arterially using iodized oil as a drug carrier, and the vessels supplying the tumor are subsequently mechanically embolized with spherical or nonspherical embolic agents. Conversely, DEB-TACE relies on the intra-arterial injection of drug-loaded microspheres that slowly release the cytotoxic drug into the tumor while at the same time embolizing its feeding vessels permanently. A less well-known TACE regimen is degradable starch microsphere (DSM) transarterial chemoembolization (DSM-TACE), a technique based on the use of degradable microspheres produced from hydrolyzed potato starch as a temporary embolic agent. What distinguishes DSM-TACE from other TACE techniques is the fact that as DSM are enzymatically degraded by blood amylases after a half-life of about 40 min (for microspheres 50 μm in diameter), the vascular occlusion obtained with this agent is transient. DSM-TACE thus combines high local drug delivery with a reduced risk of systemic toxicity while increasing the safety profile of the procedure by a short ischemia time and low vessel occlusion rate. Hence, DSM-TACE can be administered more unselectively than cTACE or DEB-TACE, making it especially suitable as a therapeutic alternative for patients with multifocal hepatic disease [1–5].

Historical Notes and Pharmacokinetics of DSM

Originally developed for scintigraphic imaging of pulmonary emboli in the early 1970s, degradable starch microspheres were found to be well tolerated when administered intravenously. Available toxicological data suggest that DSM do not directly induce any adverse reaction per se. The toxicity observed after coadministration with cytostatic agents like cisplatin, doxorubicin, or mitomycin is similar to that encountered when applying the chemotherapeutic agent alone, with the exception of enhanced liver toxicity, which is part of the desired therapeutic effect.

DSM are produced by means of polymerization from hydrolyzed potato starch, cross-linked,

T. A. Auer · F. Collettini (✉)
Charitè, Berlino, Germany

Berlin Institute of Health (BIH), Berlin, Germany
e-mail: timo-alexander.auer@charite.de; federico.collettini@charite.de

P. Lucatelli (ed.), *Transarterial Chemoembolization (TACE)*,
https://doi.org/10.1007/978-3-031-36261-3_8

and substituted with glycerol ether groups. This process results in a polymerized matrix, which has no chemical name of its own but has a complex structure well suited for transient embolization of arterial blood flow. DSM are degraded enzymatically by the body's own serum alpha-amylase. The total time of occlusion is hence indirectly proportional to the individual amount of alpha-amylase in plasma [6]. The half-life under physiological conditions at 37 °C and pH 7 ranges between 35 and 50 min. After approximately 2 h, particles are completely dissolved. The accumulating glucose monomers are dismantled and eliminated by the body's reticulocytic and excretory systems. Commercially available DSM (e.g., EmboCept® S, PharmaCept, Berlin, Germany) come in 20-ml bottles containing a sterile and clear solution consisting of 450 mg Amilomer, DSM 35/50, and 7.5 ml sodium chloride (60 mg/ml). DSM particles have a mean diameter of 50 μm with 75% of microspheres ranging in diameter from 20 to 200 μm.

8.2 Pharmacodynamics and Mechanism of Action of DSM

DSM are used to achieve blood flow reduction and transient vascular occlusion in the peritumoral blood vessels during coadministration of cytotoxic drugs. The effects of intra-arterial administration of DSM on blood flow have been investigated in numerous preclinical and clinical studies. Furthermore, several authors have explored how the altered blood flow induced by DSM affects the regional and systemic delivery of the co-injected drug.

8.2.1 DSM-Induced Blood Flow Reduction and Transient Vascular Embolization

One of the first studies investigating intra-arterial DSM was published in 1978 by Forsberg and colleagues. Forsberg et al. studied the effects of intra-arterial DSM injection into the femoral and superior mesenteric artery on blood flow in the hind feet and intestine of rats. Using tracer microspheres and electromagnetic flow measurement, they demonstrated that after DSM infusion, blood flow in the hind feet and small intestine rapidly declined to near zero and later returned to levels in control animals [6]. Thulin et al. performed preoperative electromagnetic measurement of hepatic arterial flow in 10 patients with primary or secondary liver and demonstrated that hepatic arterial blood flow could be reduced in a dose-dependent manner by a mean maximum of 67% following DSM injection [7]. Wiggermann et al. explored the transient embolizing effect of DSM-TACE using contrast-enhanced ultrasound quantitative perfusion analysis in six patients with hepatocellular carcinoma (HCC). Compared to baseline parameters, they observed a significant reduction in peak regional blood volume and regional blood flow immediately after DSM-TACE in all cases. Over time, a stepwise revascularization of the treated lesions was documented: 90 min after embolization, perfusion parameters were not significantly different from pre-embolization values [8].

A recent study addressed a central question concerning the therapeutic effect of the transient embolization achievable with DSM: Is a transient embolization sufficient to induce necrosis of the target tumor and thus inhibit its growth? Ziemann and colleagues analyzed the effect of three different agents routinely used in the setting of TACE on tumor growth in a rat model of colorectal liver metastases. The rats were randomized into four groups treated with intra-arterial infusion of either DSM (size: 35–70 μm; dose: 6.43 mg/kg body weight), PVA microspheres (size: 70–150 μm; dose: 0.14 ml/kg body weight), iodized oil (size: 2–3 μm; dose: 0.15 ml/kg body weight), or saline (control group). Tumor growth was assessed by three-dimensional ultrasound on days 8 and 11, followed by histological and immunohistochemical analysis of tumor necrosis on day 11. In this experiment, both PVA microspheres and DSM completely inhibited tumor progression while iodized oil did not significantly affect tumor growth. Immunohistochemical analysis revealed significantly larger necrotic areas within the tumors after administration of DSM and PVA microspheres compared with iodized oil [9].

8.2.2 Regional and Systemic Delivery of the co-Injected Drug

Teder et al. investigated the effects of DSM on hepatic arterial blood flow in rats by means of a regionally injected marker, ^{99m}TC-methylene diphosphonate (^{99m}Tc-MDP), and showed that compared to injections of pertechnetate only, the integrated exposure of the liver to pertechnetate was increased by a factor of 1.4–2.4 when microspheres were added [10]. In a clinical study published in 1982, Dakhil and colleagues injected DSM into the hepatic artery of patients with primary and metastatic liver cancer to assess whether transient vascular occlusion at the level of the arteriolar capillary bed would enhance regional uptake and decrease systemic exposure to simultaneously administered hepatic arterial bischlorethylnitrosourea (BCNU). Following intra-arterial DSM injection, hepatic arterial flow was transiently substantially reduced or stopped in all patients. When BCNU was given with microspheres, there was a 30–90% reduction in systemic nitrosourea exposure and in peak levels. Dakhil et al. thus demonstrated that concurrent intra-arterial injection of DSM and BCNU might have the potential to enhance selective regional drug effects while at the same time markedly reducing systemic toxicity [11]. Along this line, several authors have explored the use of DSM to increase the effectiveness of intra-arterial chemotherapy. The results of these studies show that in the presence of drastic blood flow reduction and transient vascular occlusion induced by DSM, the dwell times of co-injected drugs are prolonged within the injected area, creating a steep drug concentration gradient between the arteries and the target tissue with a selectively increased uptake of the co-injected drug into liver tumors compared with normal liver tissue [12].

8.2.3 Further Effects of DSM-Induced Transient Embolization: TACE and VEGF Expression

The combination of targeted administration of a chemotherapeutic drug at high concentration and induction of ischemia by embolization of tumor-feeding vessels is the key mechanism of TACE [13]. Local tumor hypoxia induced by TACE leads to a sequence of adaptive changes in the transcription and expression of hypoxia response genes in tumor cells aimed at counteracting or reversing hypoxia [14]. Hypoxia response genes are primarily regulated by hypoxia-inducible factor-1α (HIF-1α), which triggers expression of vascular endothelial growth factor (VEGF) and promotes neovascularization [15, 16]. Newly formed aberrant tumor blood vessels, characterized by structural and functional defects, further aggravate hypoxia and thereby form a vicious cycle thought to play a key role in tumor growth and metastatic seeding [16–18]. In the context of TACE, these biological countermeasures have the potential to interfere with the ultimate intention of anticancer treatment. In fact, studies have shown that the transient overexpression of VEGF after a single session of TACE is associated with future distant metastases, especially located in the lung or bones, and consequently with a shorter progression-free survival (PFS) [16, 19–22]. Furthermore, the peak of serum VEGF after TACE has been shown to be an independent prognostic factor of progression-fee survival (PFS) in HCC [23]. Schicho and colleagues compared serum VEGF levels in response to TACE with different embolic agents in 22 patients with HCC. In this prospective study, patients were assigned to one of three different TACE regimens (cTACE, DEB-TACE, and DSM-TACE), all performed with the same cytostatic drug (50 mg doxorubicin/m^2 body surface area (BSA)). Serum VEGF levels were assessed before TACE treatment as well as 24 h and 4 weeks after treatment. Compared to baseline, a marked increase in VEGF levels was observed 24 h after cTACE (164% of baseline level) and at 4-week follow-up (170% of baseline level). Increases in serum VEGF levels were 114% and 123% following DEB-TACE and 121% and 124% for DSM, respectively. The authors conclude that conventional TACE using Lipiodol is associated with a marked increase in blood levels of the proangiogenic factor VEGF while DEB-TACE and DSM-TACE induce only a moderate VEGF response [16].

8.3 Patients and Technique

8.3.1 Patient Selection

DSM are intended for combined use with chemotherapeutic agents to escalate effectivity by increasing the retention time of the co-injected agents in the targeted liver. Like other TACE techniques, DSM-TACE can be used in patients with primary or metastatic liver cancer not amenable to curative treatments. Regarding the treatment of hepatocellular carcinoma, guidelines from all over the world (AASLD, EASL, APASL, and ESMO) endorse the use of TACE for HCC in patients with intermediate-stage disease, defined as multinodular disease confined to the liver in asymptomatic patients (performance status of 0), Child–Pugh class A or class B cirrhosis with no decompensation, and absence of portal vein invasion or extrahepatic spread [24–27]. Absolute and relative contraindications are similar to those of cTACE and DEB-TACE and include impaired liver function, uncorrectable coagulopathies (INR >1.5; aPTT >50 s; <50,000 thrombocytes), and renal failure (serum creatinine >2 mg/dl). Relative contraindications for DSM-TACE include chronic cardiac insufficiency (NYHA III–IV), acute coronary syndrome (ACS), and exophytically growing tumors. Partial or complete thrombosis of the main portal vein is often classified as an exclusion criterion for chemoembolization. Portal vein thrombosis appears to be less of a concern for DSM-TACE due to the transient embolization and the shorter ischemia time [28].

8.3.2 DSM-TACE Technique

The goal of DSM-TACE is to achieve blood flow reduction and transient vascular occlusion in the peritumoral blood vessels to minimize systemic exposure to the co-injected cytotoxic drug. Due to the wide variation in number, size, and vascularity of liver tumors from one patient to the next, the dose of DSM has to be adapted individually. Complete stasis of blood flow should be avoided as this carries an increased risk of backflow into extrahepatic vascular territories. Hence, to perform DSM-TACE safely, angiographic monitoring during drug administration is crucial.

Angiographic techniques vary among institutions. Herein, we describe the angiographic technique as performed at our institution. In most patients, vascular access is gained through puncture of the common femoral artery in the right or left groin; however, alternative vascular access through the left radial or brachial artery may be used if this makes catheterization of the hepatic artery easier. Following arterial puncture using the Seldinger technique, a 4–/5-F angiographic sheath is introduced. After catheterization of the celiac trunk and the superior mesenteric artery using a diagnostic catheter, selective angiography of the aforementioned vessels is performed to accurately characterize the vessels supplying the liver. Subsequently, a coaxial microcatheter system is advanced beyond the branching of the gastroduodenal artery and positioned in the tumor-supplying branches of the hepatic artery. Unlike the classic TACE procedures, where the embolic agent has to be delivered as close as possible to the tumor (superselective embolization), DSM-TACE can be performed more unselectively in a lobar fashion way by placing the microcatheter in either the left or right hepatic branch. However, even for lobar administration, the use of a microcatheter is preferred to reduce the risk of vasospasm and arterial dissection. Once correct positioning of the microcatheter has been confirmed, the mixture of chemotherapeutic agent, DSM, and contrast agent is administered under constant angiographic control.

Degradable starch microspheres should be mixed with a ready-to-use solution of active substance and contrast agent. In HCC patients, DSM-TACE is performed using a mixture of 50 mg doxorubicin diluted in a saline solution with a total volume of 25 m the interval between injections to optimize the administered dose. Even if complete vascular occlusion occurs, treatment should not be discontinued, due to the risk of backflow and nontarget embolization. When DSM-TACE is performed less selectively (treatment of entire lobar or major segments), the endpoint of embolization should be a "tree-in-the-winter" appearance with occlusion of small tumor-feeding vessels but preservation of flow in the major lobar and segmental arteries. After therapy delivery, a digital subtraction angiography (DSA) is performed to confirm devascularization of target lesions and patency of the large vessels in the treated area. DSM-TACE is most effective when the procedure is performed in repeated treatment sessions. At our institution, DSM-TACE is repeated at 4- to 6-week intervals until complete disappearance of arterial enhancement is seen. In case of bilobar tumor spread in patients in whom deterioration of hepatic function is feared, the lobe with higher tumor burden is treated first, followed by the contralateral lobe. In the latter case, it is preferable to reduce the interval between the two sessions to 2 weeks if possible. Follow-up imaging is routinely performed using contrast-enhanced magnetic resonance imaging (MRI) or contrast-enhanced computed tomography (CT) in patients with contraindications to MRI.

8.4 Clinical Results and Safety

Recent experience suggests that this technique is particularly suitable for treating patients with more advanced HCC or with multifocal disease not amenable to superselective treatment [1–5]. DSM-TACE has also been tested for the palliative treatment of patients with unresectable or recurrent intrahepatic cholangiocarcinoma (iCCA) as well as for patients with chemotherapy-refractory liver metastases from colorectal cancer [29–31]. Alongside these studies, there are also reports in the literature on the use of DSM-TACE in rare entities like liver metastases from uveal melanoma, breast cancer, renal cell carcinoma, and neuroendocrine tumors [32–35].

8.4.1 Primary Liver Cancer

8.4.1.1 HCC

As already mentioned, different guidelines endorse the use of TACE in patients with intermediate-stage disease while especially DSM-TACE may also be an option in more advanced disease [3, 5, 24–27]. A recently published study by Orlacchio and colleagues evaluated the safety and efficacy of DSM-TACE in a large clinical population of 137 patients with unresectable HCC who underwent a total of 267 DSM-TACE procedures. Major complications occurred in only 6.8% of all procedures. According to mRECIST (modified Response Evaluation Criteria in Solid Tumors), a high objective response rate was obtained (84.3% of patients showed complete or partial responses), and the median time to progression was 12 months with an OS of 36 months. Of note, 20 patients in the study had BCLC stage C HCC [36]. In another recently published study, Iezzi and colleagues investigated DSM-TACE treatment in 40 consecutive BCLC stage B or C patients with intermediate or locally advanced stage HCC who dismissed or were ineligible for sorafenib. While technical success was achieved in all patients, no liver failure or systemic toxicity was reported. Progression-free survival (PFS) was 6.4 months and the median OS was 11.3 months [3]. These results have been corroborated in a study of *Haubold and colleagues*, who investigated DSM-TACE in non-resectable HCC patients ineligible for other systemic or locoregional therapies. DSM-TACE was performed successfully in 28 patients. At control imaging after three DSM-TACE procedures, the rates of complete response (CR), partial response (PR), stable disease (SD), and progressive disease (PD) were 14.3%, 25%, 39.3%, and 21.4%, respectively. With a good OS of 682 days, the authors also conclude that DSM-TACE is a safe and promising treatment alternative. A selection of further studies in line with the results just outlined is provided in the table below (Table 8.1) [1–5, 36–41].

8.4.1.2 Intrahepatic Cholangiocarcinoma

Intrahepatic cholangiocarcinoma (iCCA) is the second most common primary liver malignancy after hepatocellular carcinoma, and its incidence and mortality have risen globally in the past decades [42]. Despite substantial advances in diagnosis and treatment, the prognosis of patients with iCCA remains poor [42]. This is mainly due to the fact that at the time of initial diagnosis, only about 20% of patients are amenable to surgical resection, the only potentially curative treatment option for iCCA [43]. Despite a low level of evidence, locoregional therapies have shown promising results in the treatment of selected patients with unresectable or recurrent disease [44]. TACE of iCCA has been investigated in several, mostly retrospective, studies using various chemotherapeutic agents. In a recently published systematic meta-analysis of 13 studies (906 patients), pooled median survival after TACE was 14.2 months [45].

Two studies on the use of DSM-TACE in patients with unresectable iCCA have been published. Georg et al. reported their experience with a multi-agent (cisplatin/doxorubicin/mitomycin C) DSM-TACE protocol in a population of 21 patients with either unresectable iCCA progressive under systemic chemotherapy or unresectable intrahepatic tumor recurrence after prior major liver resection. The reported objective response rate was 61.1% and the reported disease control rate 100%. Median overall survival was 13.3 months with similar results in patients with primary unresectable, therapy-refractory disease (13.2 months) and patients with intrahepatic recurrence after prior liver resection (12.5 months) (Table 8.2) [30].

8.4.2 Secondary Liver Cancer

8.4.2.1 Colorectal Cancer Liver Metastasis

Colorectal cancer (CRC) is one of the most common cancers worldwide, ranking third in terms of incidence and second in terms of cancer-related death [46]. The liver is the most common site of colorectal cancer metastasis. Approximately 20% of patients with CRC present with concomitant liver metastasis at initial diagnosis while another 50% develop liver metastasis within the first 3 years after diagnosis [47]. Surgery offers the best chance of cure for patients with colorectal liver metastases (CRLM); however, only 10–25% of all patients with CRLM are amenable to surgical resection [48]. Locoregional treatments have proven to be a useful therapeutic strategy in patients with unresectable CRLM. TACE has been identified as a suitable treatment option for patients with CRLM in a neoadjuvant, symptomatic, or palliative setting [31, 49–53]. One of the first studies investigating the use of DSM-TACE in the management of CRLM was published in 2013 by Nishiofuku and colleagues. The authors reported the results of a phase I/II trial of DSM-TACE with cisplatin powder in 24 patients with unresectable CRLM progressing after FOLFOX (5-flourouracil, leucovorin plus oxaliplatin) chemotherapy. In phase II, the tumor response rate was 61.1%, and median overall survival was 21.1 months [54]. In a recent prospective, randomized, single-center trial, Vogl et al. com-

Table 8.1 Most important publications on DSM-TACE therapy in HCC of the past decade

Authors (year)	n	Design	Aim	Conclusion/major results
Minici et al. (2021)	50	Single center Retrospective	Safety and efficacy of DSM-TACE in BCLC B HCC in patients with a child-Pugh score of 8–9	DSM-TACE is effective and safe in intermediate-stage HCC, achieving an interesting downstaging rate.
Vogl et al. (2021)	61	Single center Prospective	cTACE vs. cTACE + DSM-TACE in BCLC B stage HCC based on metric tumor response and survival	cTACE + DSM-TACE showed a significant benefit in tumor response compared to cTACE only but no benefit in survival time.
Auer et al. (2020)	36	Single center Retrospective	DSM-TACE vs. SIRT in multifocal HCC based on survival rates and side effects	DSM-TACE = OS/PFS: 4 months SIRT = OS/PFS: 6 months DSM-TACE might be an alternative to SIRT in multifocal HCC.
Haubold et al. (2020)	28	Single center Retrospective	DSM-TACE of HCC: Evaluation of tumor response in patients ineligible for other systemic or locoregional therapies	CR: 14.3%; PR: 25%; SD: 39.3%; PD: 21.4% DSM-TACE is a safe and promising treatment alternative.
Gross et al. (2020)	37	Single center Retrospective	DSM-TACE and anthracyclines in patients with locally extensive HCC: Safety and efficacy	Median OS: 19 m (BCLC B: 22 m BCLC C/D: 6.7 m) DSM-TACE of HCC is safe even in patients with advanced disease.
Iezzi et al. (2019)	40	Single center Retrospective	DSM-TACE as second-line treatment in HCC patients dismissing or ineligible for sorafenib	PFS: 6.4 m/OS: 11.3 DSM-TACE is a safe and effective second-line treatment in patients ineligible for sorafenib.
Orlacchio et al. (2018)	137	Single center Retrospective	Safety and efficacy of DSM-TACE in a large clinical patient population with unresectable HCC	84.3% of patients showed CR or PR. DSM-TACE is a safe and effective therapy for patients with HCC, allowing to obtain a good rate of OS with excellent local tumor control.
Gruber-Rouh et al. (2018)	99	Single center Retrospective	cTACE vs. cTACE + DSM-TACE in HCC based on metric tumor response and survival	No significant difference between TACE regimens investigated.
Orlacchio et al. (2018)	24	Single center Prospective	Safety and response rates of DSM-TACE in patients with unresectable HCC	20.8% CR. DSM-TACE is a valid, well-tolerated alternative treatment to Lipiodol-TACE or DEB-TACE.
Schicho et al. (2017)	179	Multicenter Retrospective	Safety and efficacy of DSM-TACE in HCC	CR: 2%; PR: 42% SD: 26%; PD: 18% *"The use of DSM as a TACE embolic agent appears to be safe for the treatment of HCC and has promising efficacy."*
Niessen et al. (2013)	69	Single center Retrospective	To compare outcomes of cTACE vs. DSM-TACE in intermediate-stage HCC	DSM-TACE is an alternative method of HCC treatment compared to cTACE.

Table 8.2 Most important studies of DSM-TACE in the treatment of iCC

Authors (year)	n	Design	Aim	Conclusion/major results
Georg et al. (2019)	21	Single center Retrospective	Efficacy and complication rates of DSM-TACE in unresectable iCC	DSM-TACE is an effective treatment for unresectable and otherwise therapy-refractory iCC.
Schicho et al. (2017)	7	Multicenter Retrospective	Safety and efficacy of DSM-TACE in the treatment of iCC	44% disease control. The use of DSM as an embolic agent for TACE is safe in the treatment of ICC.

Table 8.3 Most important studies of DSM-TACE in the treatment of CRLM

Authors (year)	n	Design	Aim	Conclusion/major results
Vogl et al. (2021)	31	Single center Prospective Randomized	To evaluate the therapy response of third-line TACE with DSM or Lipiodol in the treatment of CRLM using MRI	DSM-TACE achieved significantly better outcomes than cTACE in terms of tumor volume reduction and tumor response according to RECIST 1.1.
Gruber-Rouh et al. (2014)	564	Single center Retrospective	To evaluate the therapeutic efficacy in patients with CRC liver metastases treated with TACE (DSM-TACE i.a.)	TACE is a therapy option for controlling local metastases and improving survival time in patients with hepatic metastases from CRC.
Nishiofuku et al. (2013)	24	Phase I/II single-center, single-arm, open-label trial	Determination of the recommended cisplatin powder dose and assessment of the efficacy and safety of the procedure	DSM-TACE with cisplatin powder at a dose of 80 mg/m^2 is well tolerated and can produce a high response rate with a long survival time for patients with unresectable CRLM after failure of FOLFOX.

pared the therapy response of third-line cTACE (n = 13) versus DSM-TACE (n = 18) in 31 patients with CRLM. In this first prospective study directly comparing cTACE and DSM-TACE in patients with CRLM, DSM-TACE showed significantly better results in terms of tumor volume reduction (p = 0.006) and tumor response according to RECIST 1.1 (p = 0.047) compared with cTACE [31]. Please find a list of studies in Table 8.3 [31, 49, 54].

Other Entities

Experience with DSM-TACE in the treatment of other entities is based on relatively limited single-center experiences; a selection of studies is compiled in Table 8.4 [33, 55–59].

Table 8.4 Most important studies of DSM-TACE alone or as additive treatment or in combination with other therapies in the treatment of liver metastases from different primaries

Authors	n	Design	Aim	Conclusion/major results
Lindgaard et al. (2018)	52	Bicentric, prospective (phase II trial)	HAT (DSM-TACE i.a.) for liver metastases in patients with metastatic breast cancer	HAT oxaliplatin in combination with capecitabine (+DSM-TACE) is safe and efficient in patients with breast cancer liver metastases.
Eichler et al. (2013)	43	Single center Prospective Non-randomized (phase II trial)	Efficacy in patients with inoperable liver metastases from breast cancer	DSM-TACE with gemcitabine is well tolerated and provides an alternative treatment for patients with liver metastases from breast cancer.
Vogl et al. (2012)	56	Single center Retrospective	To evaluate the local tumor control and survival data after TACE with different drug combinations (DSM-TACE among i.a.) in the palliative treatment of patients with liver metastases from gastric cancer	Transarterial chemoembolization is a minimally invasive therapy option for palliative treatment of liver metastases in patients with gastric cancer.
Azizi et al. (2011)	32	Single center Retrospective	Effect of chemoembolization on **pancreatic cancer** liver metastases	Repetitive TACE resulted in a relevant response for the control of pancreatic cancer liver metastases with respectable median survival time.
Vogl et al. (2011)	65	Single center Retrospective	Local tumor control and survival data after TACE (DSM-TACE i.a.) as third-line treatment of patients with ovarian cancer liver metastases	TACE is an effective palliative treatment in achieving local control in selected patients with liver metastases from ovarian cancer.
Nabil et al. (2008)	22	Single center Retrospective	Effectiveness of TACE with Lipiodol and DSM in local tumor control and survival in patients with hepatic metastases from renal cell carcinoma	TACE can result in a favorable local tumor response in patients with hepatic metastases from RCC, but survival results are still limited.

8.5 Conclusions

- DSM is a short-acting, nonpermanent embolic agent and therefore can be administered unselectively.
- DSM-TACE is a safe and easy to perform interventional procedure and a useful therapeutic alternative for patients with multifocal HCC.
- Other indications for DSM-TACE are neoadjuvant, symptomatic, and palliative treatment of locally extensive or disseminated ICC or CRLM.
- While DSM-TACE should be suitable for nearly any patient with disseminated metastatic liver disease, evidence is still limited, except for CRLM, and published data are mostly based on monocentric studies with limited patient numbers.

References

1. Auer TA, Jonczyk M, Collettini F, Marth A, Wieners G, Hamm B, et al. Trans-arterial chemoembolization with degradable starch microspheres (DSM-TACE) versus selective internal radiation therapy (SIRT) in multifocal hepatocellular carcinoma. Acta Radiol. 2021;62(3):313–21.
2. Haubold J, Reinboldt MP, Wetter A, Li Y, Ludwig JM, Lange C, et al. DSM-TACE of HCC: evaluation of tumor response in patients ineligible for other systemic or loco-regional therapies. RoFo: Fortschritte auf dem Gebiete der Rontgenstrahlen und der Nuklearmedizin. 2020;192(9):862–9.
3. Iezzi R, Pompili M, Rinninella E, Annicchiarico E, Garcovich M, Cerrito L, et al. TACE with degradable starch microspheres (DSM-TACE) as second-line treatment in HCC patients dismissing or ineligible for sorafenib. Eur Radiol. 2019;29(3):1285–92.
4. Schicho A, Pereira PL, Haimerl M, Niessen C, Michalik K, Beyer LP, et al. Transarterial chemoembolization (TACE) with degradable starch microspheres (DSM) in hepatocellular carcinoma (HCC): multi-center results on safety and efficacy. Oncotarget. 2017;8(42):72613–20.
5. Gross A, Albrecht T. Transarterial chemoembolisation (TACE) with degradable starch microspheres (DSM) and anthracycline in patients with locally extensive hepatocellular carcinoma (HCC): safety and efficacy. Cardiovasc Intervent Radiol. 2020;43(3):402–10.
6. Forsberg JO. Transient blood flow reduction induced by intra-arterial injection of degradable starch microspheres. Experiments on rats. Acta Chir Scand. 1978;144(5):275–81.
7. Thulin L, Tyden G, Nyberg B, Calissendorff B, Hultcrantz R. Reduction of hepatic arterial flow by degradable microspheres in patients with liver tumor. Acta Chir Scand. 1986;152:447–51.
8. Wiggermann P, Wohlgemuth WA, Heibl M, Vasilj A, Loss M, Schreyer AG, et al. Dynamic evaluation and quantification of microvascularization during degradable starch microspheres transarterial chemoembolisation (DSM-TACE) of HCC lesions using contrast enhanced ultrasound (CEUS): a feasibility study. Clin Hemorheol Microcirc. 2013;53(4):337–48.
9. Ziemann C, Roller J, Malter MM, Keller K, Kollmar O, Glanemann M, et al. Intra-arterial EmboCept S(R) and DC bead(R) effectively inhibit tumor growth of colorectal rat liver metastases. BMC Cancer. 2019;19(1):938.
10. Teder H, Nilsson M, Aronsen KF, Erichsen C, Jonsson PE. Influence of degradable starch microspheres (Spherex) on the retention of pertechnetate in a solitary rat liver tumor. European J Surg Oncol. 1988;14(4):327–33.
11. Dakhil S, Ensminger W, Cho K, Niederhuber J, Doan K, Wheeler R. Improved regional selectivity of hepatic arterial BCNU with degradable microspheres. Cancer. 1982;50(4):631–5.
12. Civalleri D, Esposito M, Fulco RA, Vannozzi M, Balletto N, De Cian F, et al. Liver and tumor uptake and plasma pharmacokinetic of arterial cisplatin administered with and without starch microspheres in patients with liver metastases. Cancer. 1991;68(5):988–94.
13. Llovet JM, Real MI, Montaña X, Planas R, Coll S, Aponte J, et al. Arterial embolisation or chemoembolisation versus symptomatic treatment in patients with unresectable hepatocellular carcinoma: a randomised controlled trial. Lancet. 2002;359(9319):1734–9.
14. Carmeliet P. Angiogenesis in life, disease and medicine. Nature. 2005;438(7070):932–6.
15. Span PN, Bussink J. Biology of hypoxia. Seminars in nuclear medicine. Elsevier; 2015.
16. Schicho A, Hellerbrand C, Kruger K, Beyer LP, Wohlgemuth W, Niessen C, et al. Impact of different embolic agents for Transarterial chemoembolization (TACE) procedures on systemic vascular endothelial growth factor (VEGF) levels. J Clin Transl Hepatol. 2016;4(4):288–92.
17. Miura H, Miyazaki T, Kuroda M, Oka T, Machinami R, Kodama T, et al. Increased expression of vascular endothelial growth factor in human hepatocellular carcinoma. J Hepatol. 1997;27(5):854–61.
18. Yamaguchi R, Yano H, Iemura A, Ogasawara S, Haramaki M, Kojiro M. Expression of vascular endothelial growth factor in human hepatocellular carcinoma. Hepatology. 1998;28(1):68–77.
19. Li X, Feng GS, Zheng CS, Zhuo CK, Liu X. Expression of plasma vascular endothelial growth factor in patients with hepatocellular carcinoma and effect of transcatheter arterial chemoembolization

therapy on plasma vascular endothelial growth factor level. World J Gastroenterol. 2004;10(19):2878–82.
20. Poon RT, Lau C, Yu WC, Fan ST, Wong J. High serum levels of vascular endothelial growth factor predict poor response to transarterial chemoembolization in hepatocellular carcinoma: a prospective study. Oncol Rep. 2004;11(5):1077–84.
21. Xiong ZP, Yang SR, Liang ZY, Xiao EH, Yu XP, Zhou SK, et al. Association between vascular endothelial growth factor and metastasis after transcatheter arterial chemoembolization in patients with hepatocellular carcinoma. Zhonghua Zhong Liu Za Zhi. 2004;3(3):386–90.
22. Sergio A, Cristofori C, Cardin R, Pivetta G, Ragazzi R, Baldan A, et al. Transcatheter arterial chemoembolization (TACE) in hepatocellular carcinoma (HCC): the role of angiogenesis and invasiveness. Am J Gastroenterol. 2008;103(4):914–21.
23. Shim JH, Park JW, Kim JH, An M, Kong SY, Nam BH, et al. Association between increment of serum VEGF level and prognosis after transcatheter arterial chemoembolization in hepatocellular carcinoma patients. Cancer Sci. 2008;99(10):2037–44.
24. European Association for the Study of the Liver. Electronic address eee, European Association for the Study of the L. EASL clinical practice guidelines: management of hepatocellular carcinoma. J Hepatol. 2018;69(1):182–236.
25. Marrero JA, Kulik LM, Sirlin CB, Zhu AX, Finn RS, Abecassis MM, et al. Diagnosis, staging, and Management of Hepatocellular Carcinoma: 2018 practice guidance by the American Association for the Study of Liver Diseases. Hepatology. 2018;68(2):723–50.
26. Omata M, Cheng AL, Kokudo N, Kudo M, Lee JM, Jia J, et al. Asia-Pacific clinical practice guidelines on the management of hepatocellular carcinoma: a 2017 update. Hepatol Int. 2017;11(4):317–70.
27. Vogel A, Cervantes A, Chau I, Daniele B, Llovet JM, Meyer T, et al. Hepatocellular carcinoma: ESMO Clinical Practice Guidelines for diagnosis, treatment and follow-up. Ann Oncol. 2018;29(Suppl 4):iv238–iv55.
28. Lucatelli P, Burrel M, Guiu B, de Rubeis G, van Delden O, Helmberger T. CIRSE standards of practice on hepatic Transarterial chemoembolisation. Cardiovasc Intervent Radiol. 2021;44(12):1851–67.
29. Schicho A, Pereira PL, Putzler M, Michalik K, Albrecht T, Nolte-Ernsting C, et al. Degradable starch microspheres Transcatheter arterial chemoembolization (DSM-TACE) in intrahepatic Cholangiocellular carcinoma (ICC): results from a National Multi-Center Study on safety and efficacy. Med Sci Monit. 2017;23:796–800.
30. Goerg F, Zimmermann M, Bruners P, Neumann U, Luedde T, Kuhl C. Chemoembolization with degradable starch microspheres for treatment of patients with primary or recurrent Unresectable, locally advanced intrahepatic cholangiocarcinoma: a pilot study. Cardiovasc Intervent Radiol. 2019;42(12):1709–17.
31. Vogl TJ, Marko C, Langenbach MC, Naguib NNN, Filmann N, Hammerstingl R, et al. Transarterial chemoembolization of colorectal cancer liver metastasis: improved tumor response by DSM-TACE versus conventional TACE, a prospective, randomized, single-center trial. Eur Radiol. 2021;31(4):2242–51.
32. Schuster R, Lindner M, Wacker F, Krossin M, Bechrakis N, Foerster MH, et al. Transarterial chemoembolization of liver metastases from uveal melanoma after failure of systemic therapy: toxicity and outcome. Melanoma Res. 2010;20(3):191–6.
33. Nabil M, Gruber T, Yakoub D, Ackermann H, Zangos S, Vogl TJ. Repetitive transarterial chemoembolization (TACE) of liver metastases from renal cell carcinoma: local control and survival results. Eur Radiol. 2008;18(7):1456–63.
34. Vogl TJ, Gruber T, Naguib NN, Hammerstingl R, Nour-Eldin NE. Liver metastases of neuroendocrine tumors: treatment with hepatic transarterial chemotherapy using two therapeutic protocols. AJR Am J Roentgenol. 2009;193(4):941–7.
35. Schneider P, Foitzik T, Pohlen U, Golder W, Buhr HJ. Temporary unilateral microembolization of the lung-a new approach to regional chemotherapy for pulmonary metastases. J Surg Res. 2002;107(2):159–66.
36. Orlacchio A, Chegai F, Roma S, Merolla S, Bosa A, Francioso S. Degradable starch microspheres transarterial chemoembolization (DSMs-TACE) in patients with unresectable hepatocellular carcinoma (HCC): long-term results from a single-center 137-patient cohort prospective study. Radiol Med. 2020;125(1):98–106.
37. Orlacchio A, Chegai F, Francioso S, Merolla S, Monti S, Angelico M, et al. Repeated Transarterial chemoembolization with degradable starch microspheres (DSMs-TACE) of Unresectable hepatocellular carcinoma: a prospective pilot study. Curr Med Imaging Rev. 2018;14(4):637–45.
38. Niessen C, Unterpaintner E, Goessmann H, Schlitt HJ, Mueller-Schilling M, Wohlgemuth WA, et al. Degradable starch microspheres versus ethiodol and doxorubicin in transarterial chemoembolization of hepatocellular carcinoma. J Vasc Interv Radiol. 2014;25(2):240–7.
39. Vogl TJ, Langenbach MC, Hammerstingl R, Albrecht MH, Chatterjee AR, Gruber-Rouh T. Evaluation of two different transarterial chemoembolization protocols using Lipiodol and degradable starch microspheres in therapy of hepatocellular carcinoma: a prospective trial. Hepatol Int. 2021;15:685.
40. Gruber-Rouh T, Schmitt C, Naguib NNN, Nour-Eldin NA, Eichler K, Beeres M, et al. Transarterial chemoembolization (TACE) using mitomycin and lipiodol with or without degradable starch microspheres for hepatocellular carcinoma: comparative study. BMC Cancer. 2018;18(1):188.
41. Minici R, Ammendola M, Manti F, Siciliano MA, Giglio E, Minici M, et al. Safety and efficacy of degradable starch microspheres Transcatheter arterial chemoembolization as a bridging therapy in patients

with early stage hepatocellular carcinoma and child-Pugh stage B eligible for liver transplant. Front Pharmacol. 2021;12:634084.

42. Valle JW, Kelley RK, Nervi B, Oh DY, Zhu AX. Biliary tract cancer. Lancet. 2021;397(10272):428–44.
43. Ebata T, Ercolani G, Alvaro D, Ribero D, Di Tommaso L, Valle JW. Current status on cholangiocarcinoma and gallbladder cancer. Liver Cancer. 2016;6(1):59–65.
44. Fabritius MP, Ben Khaled N, Kunz WG, Ricke J, Seidensticker M. Image-guided local treatment for Unresectable intrahepatic cholangiocarcinoma-role of interventional radiology. J Clin Med. 2021;10(23)
45. Mosconi C, Solaini L, Vara G, Brandi N, Cappelli A, Modestino F, et al. Transarterial chemoembolization and Radioembolization for Unresectable intrahepatic cholangiocarcinoma—a systemic review and meta-analysis. Cardiovasc Intervent Radiol. 2021;1-11:728.
46. Bray F, Ferlay J, Soerjomataram I, Siegel RL, Torre LA, Jemal A. Global cancer statistics 2018: GLOBOCAN estimates of incidence and mortality worldwide for 36 cancers in 185 countries. CA Cancer J Clin. 2018;68(6):394–424.
47. Tasoudis PT, Ziogas IA, Alexopoulos SP, Fung JJ, Tsoulfas G. Role of liver transplantation in the management of colorectal liver metastases: challenges and opportunities. World J Clin Oncol. 2021;12(12):1193–201.
48. Sasson AR, Sigurdson ER. Surgical treatment of liver metastases. Semin Oncol. 2002;29(2):107–18.
49. Gruber-Rouh T, Naguib NN, Eichler K, Ackermann H, Zangos S, Trojan J, et al. Transarterial chemoembolization of unresectable systemic chemotherapy-refractory liver metastases from colorectal cancer: long-term results over a 10-year period. Int J Cancer. 2014;134(5):1225–31.
50. Mahnken AH, Pereira PL, de Baere T. Interventional oncologic approaches to liver metastases. Radiology. 2013;266(2):407–30.
51. Clark TW. Chemoembolization for colorectal liver metastases after FOLFOX failure. J Vasc Interv Radiol. 2013;24(1):66–7.
52. Gruber-Rouh T, Marko C, Thalhammer A, Nour-Eldin NE, Langenbach M, Beeres M, et al. Current strategies in interventional oncology of colorectal liver metastases. Br J Radiol. 2016;89(1064):20151060.
53. Wasser K, Giebel F, Fischbach R, Tesch H, Landwehr P. Transarterial chemoembolization of liver metastases of colorectal carcinoma using degradable starch microspheres (Spherex): personal investigations and review of the literature. Radiologe. 2005;45(7):633–43.
54. Nishiofuku H, Tanaka T, Matsuoka M, Otsuji T, Anai H, Sueyoshi S, et al. Transcatheter arterial chemoembolization using cisplatin powder mixed with degradable starch microspheres for colorectal liver metastases after FOLFOX failure: results of a phase I/II study. J Vasc Interv Radiol. 2013;24(1):56–65.
55. Lindgaard SC, Brinch CM, Jensen BK, Norgaard HH, Hermann KL, Theile S, et al. Hepatic arterial therapy with oxaliplatin and systemic capecitabine for patients with liver metastases from breast cancer. Breast. 2019;43:113–9.
56. Eichler K, Jakobi S, Gruber-Rouh T, Hammerstingl R, Vogl TJ, Zangos S. Transarterial chemoembolisation (TACE) with gemcitabine: phase II study in patients with liver metastases of breast cancer. Eur J Radiol. 2013;82(12):e816–22.
57. Vogl TJ, Gruber-Rouh T, Eichler K, Nour-Eldin NE, Trojan J, Zangos S, et al. Repetitive transarterial chemoembolization (TACE) of liver metastases from gastric cancer: local control and survival results. Eur J Radiol. 2013;82(2):258–63.
58. Azizi A, Naguib NN, Mbalisike E, Farshid P, Emami AH, Vogl TJ. Liver metastases of pancreatic cancer: role of repetitive transarterial chemoembolization (TACE) on tumor response and survival. Pancreas. 2011;40(8):1271–5.
59. Vogl TJ, Naguib NN, Lehnert T, Nour-Eldin NE, Eichler K, Zangos S, et al. Initial experience with repetitive transarterial chemoembolization (TACE) as a third line treatment of ovarian cancer metastasis to the liver: indications, outcomes and role in patient's management. Gynecol Oncol. 2012;124(2):225–9.

Balloon-Occluded TACE 9

Pierleone Lucatelli, Fabrizio Basilico, Bianca Rocco, and Carlo Catalano

Balloon-occluded TACE (b-TACE) is a transarterial chemoembolization in which the microcatheter used to deliver the chemotherapy and embolizing material has a micro-balloon at its distal end.

By inflating the micro-balloon, a temporary block flow can be performed within the tributary feeder of the target lesion, which allows redistribution of flow within the area to be treated (Fig. 9.1).

The first TACE procedure using a balloon catheter was described by Nakamura in 1991 in order to prevent embolization of gastric vessels [1], but it was Irie in 2013 who applied to chemoembolization the "balloon-assisted" technique [2]. Over the years, this technique has been applied in conventional TACE (C-b-TACE, performed with Lipiodol emulsion and chemotherapeutic drug) and recently in drug-eluting microsphere TACE (DEM-b-TACE) [3]. Since no significant differences were demonstrated, either in tumor response or overall survival, between the aforementioned procedures, the choice of embolization technique mostly relies on operator preference.

In a recent study, Rose et al. [4] compared the results of tumor response rate and mean dose of drug or emulsion delivered in patients undergoing TACE with and without "balloon-assisted technique" and found significantly higher mean dose of drug or emulsion delivered using b-TACE procedure. These results were confirmed by Lucatelli et al. [5] who evaluated the role of the balloon microcatheter in vivo comparing b-DEB-TACE vs. DEB-TACE and b-SIRT vs. SIRT. Among the two DEB-TACE groups, the balloon microcatheter-treated groups showed significantly higher contrast, signal-to-noise ratio, and contrast-to-noise ratio when compared to conventional DEB-TACE; analyzing the two SIRT groups, instead, 2D dosimetry profile evaluation showed an activity intensity peak significantly higher in the b-SIRT than in the SIRT subgroup. Moreover, in histological explanted liver analysis, there was a trend for higher intratumoral localization of embolic microspheres for b-DEB-TACE in comparison with DEB-TACE. The results of this study demonstrate, in vivo, a better embolization profile of oncological intra-arterial interventions performed with balloon microcatheter regardless of the embolic agent employed. The same group published a case control study to compare oncological results and safety profile of b-DEB-TACE in patients with hepatocellular carcinoma [6]. This study showed a trend of better oncological response over DEM-TACE, with a longer time to retreat interval, and a similar adverse events rate, in patients presenting with larger tumors.

P. Lucatelli (✉) · F. Basilico · B. Rocco · C. Catalano
Vascular and Interventional Radiology Unit, Department of Radiological, Oncological, and Anatomo-Pathological Sciences, Sapienza University of Rome, Rome, Italy

P. Lucatelli (ed.), *Transarterial Chemoembolization (TACE)*,
https://doi.org/10.1007/978-3-031-36261-3_9

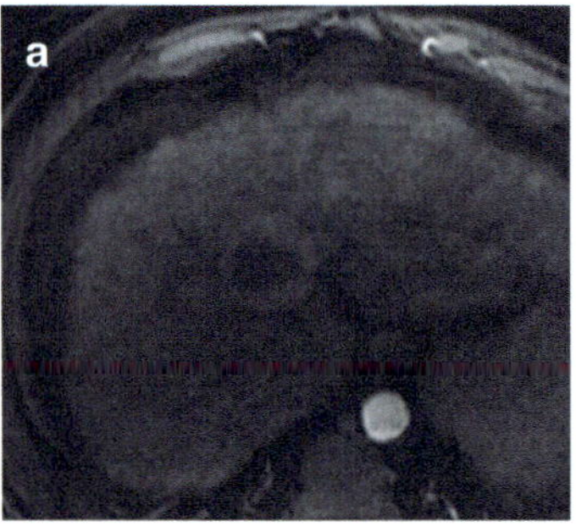

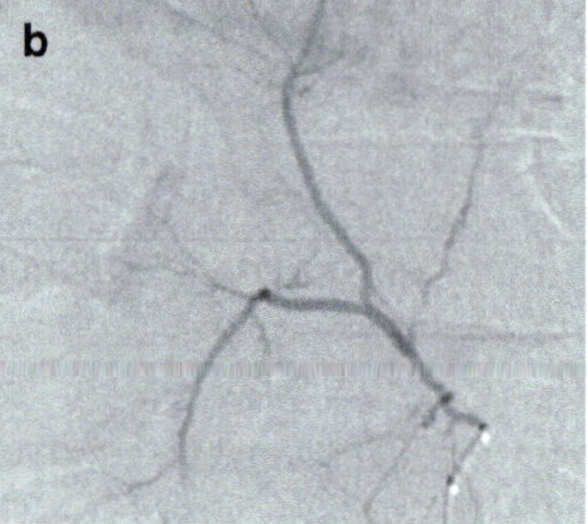

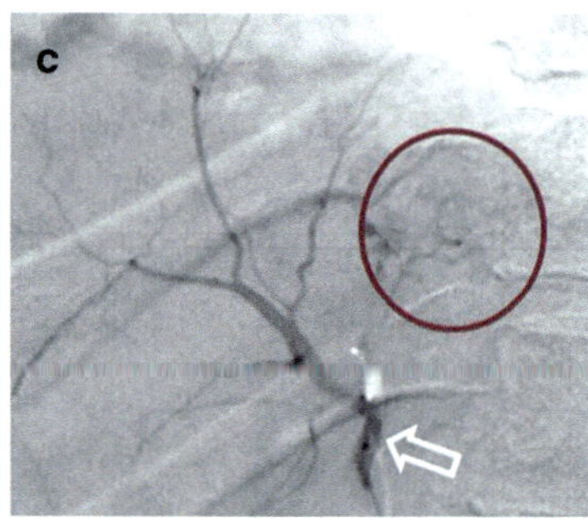

Fig. 9.1 Hepatocarcinoma of the IV segment with hypervascular rim in arterial phase on preprocedural MRI (**a**). Selective angiography performed from the microcatheter with a deflated micro-balloon (**b**) does not depict the lesion, which appears appreciable after micro-balloon inflation (**c**) due to the redistribution of flow toward the tumor lesion

The oncological performance of the TACE, both with its application in the conventional approach and in DEE-TACE, was proven to be ameliorated by micro-balloon employment. A better therapeutic effect ($p = 0.016$) and improved control rates of the primary nodule ($p = 0.0016$) were proved in a study by Irie et al. [7]. The same study showed no statistically significant differences in overall survival or tumor-free rates in the liver. The largest European multicentric study [8] proved a higher complete response rate in the treatment of 30–50 mm HCC ($p = 0.047$), as well as a significantly lower retreatment rate after a single TACE in comparison with cTACE (12.1% vs. 26.9%, respectively; $p = 0.005$).

Overall survival rates ranged from 89.6% to 85.7% at 1 year, from 57.3% to 52.3% at 2 years, and from 46.7% to 17.1% at 3 years [9–11].

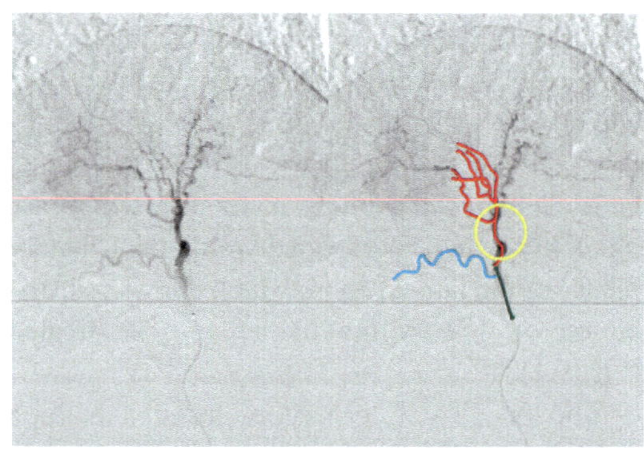

Fig. 9.2 The identification of the vessel in which to inflate the micro-balloon is a crucial decision in b-TACE. A straight segment of vessel (green) must be selected, avoiding tortuous segments (yellow). The presence of the micro-balloon ensures that "nontarget" branches are occluded (blue) and at the same time provides a good vascular territory downstream for redistribution of flow to the lesion (red)

9.1 Microcatheter Positioning and Inflation

In b-TACE, it is essential to obtain a detailed mapping of the arterial vasculature (cone-beam CT) in order to identify the best vascular segment where to inflate the micro-balloon.

CBCT acquisition should preferably be biphasic and performed through a 4-Fr diagnostic catheter, possibly placed before the bifurcation of the hepatic artery in its right and left branches. This is particularly important for lesions located in "watershed" segments (e.g., segments IV and V–VIII). The CBCT acquisition is usually performed with a single bolus of contrast diluted at 30%, with a flow rate between 3 and 4 ml/s for a duration of 15 s, necessary to cover the time required to perform the first rotation of the C-arm (between 5 and 12 s depending on the type of angiography system). Using the MPR and 3D reconstructions obtained from the CBCT datasets, it is possible to identify the number and provenience of the feeders of the target lesions. The microcatheter should be placed in as straight a vascular segment as possible, proximal to all target lesions to maximize the effectiveness [12] (Fig. 9.2). If there are feeders that cannot be occluded and are in competition with the primary

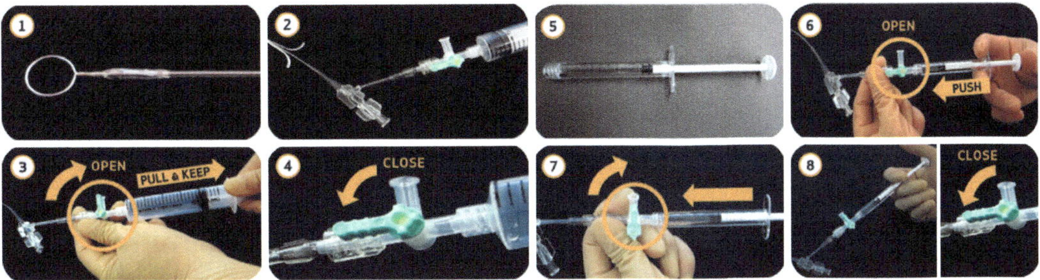

Fig. 9.3 Priming of the Occlusafe microcatheter: (1) distal end of microcatheter with stiletto; (2,3,4) vacuum (for approximately 10 s) of the micro-balloon using a 10-ml Luer-lock syringe and subsequently closing the balloon lumen; (5,6,7,8) preparation for inflation of the micro-balloon using a 1-ml graduated syringe

feeder, the effectiveness in determining redistribution may be suboptimal.

Before using the microcatheter, it is necessary to do a correct "priming" of the balloon inflation line. This consists of aspiration of the lateral lumen of the micro-balloon to remove any residual air and verify its structural integrity (Fig. 9.3). For optimal results, the following steps are recommended:

1. Using a three-way valve and Luer-lock syringes (10-cc syringes), vacuum is applied to the inflation channel.
2. To check for correct integrity, the syringe included in the kit must be connected to the micro-balloon route and loaded with a diluted contrast media solution (50–70% saline).
3. If the vacuum procedure has been correctly performed, after opening the three-way valve, an automatic aspiration of the syringe volume corresponding to the volume needed to fill the dead space of the balloon channel will be observed.
4. Once the syringe plunger has stopped, we are ready to inject the amount of volume required to inflate the micro-balloon and make it adhere to the vessel wall.

Prior to use, it is necessary to verify the integrity of the device, as well as to allow the operator to understand the latency time that must be waited during the inflation in vivo to see the inflated micro-balloon in the angiography system (typically 20 s). In order to evaluate and control the appropriate inflation of the micro-balloon, it is important to carefully assess the size of the arterial feeder and to continuously evaluate the arterial pressure measured at the tip of the microcatheter.

Size of the feeder assessment is crucial because the balloon can be distended to 2, 3, and 4 mm, injecting 0.04, 0.06, and 0.1 ml of inflation solution, respectively. Excessive stretching in small vessels may be associated with damage to the vessel wall. In vessels greater than 4 mm in diameter, it will not be possible to bring the balloon into contact with the arterial walls, thus not allowing the pressure drop that triggers flow redistribution.

Inflation of the balloon should be performed very slowly, injecting the inflation solution (typically contrast media and saline in a 60:40 ratio) with the 1-ml syringe available in the kit. It is recommended to pay attention to respect the inflation volumes indicated by the manufacturer, more than to the visual confirmation in the monitor: a latency time of about 20 s from the injection to the actual inflation of the balloon is appreciable, which may lead to overfilling of the balloon (even to rupture) in case of exceeding the injected volume.

Arterial pressure can be measured using a simple closed-circuit kit and a pressure transducer, connected directly to a monitor normally used for invasive blood pressure measurement. This method of measurement allows you to evaluate both the pressure wave and the numerical value (Fig. 9.4).

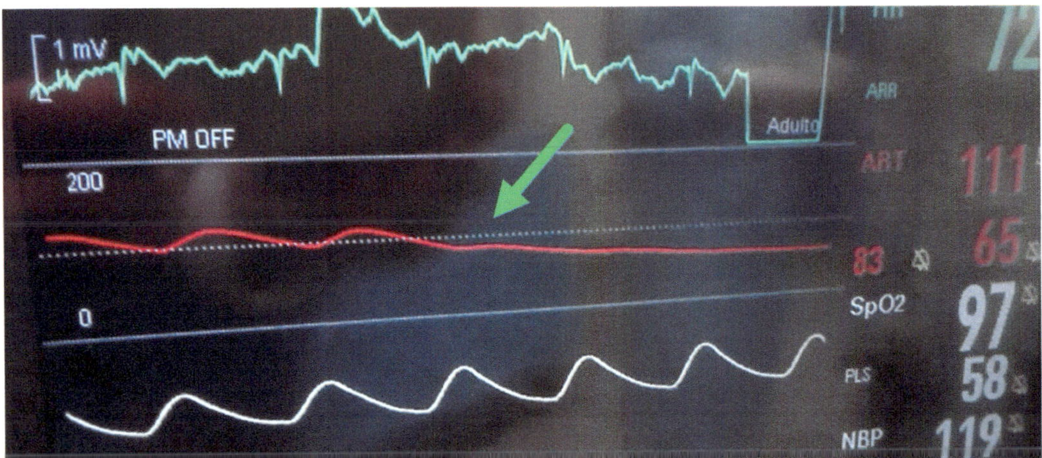

Fig. 9.4 A pressure transducer connected to a monitor using a closed-circuit kit normally used for invasive blood pressure measurement. After inflation of the micro-balloon, a flattening of the pressure wave curve is observed with a consensual decrease in the numerical value of the average pressure

An initial invasive pressure measurement is taken, which must be compatible with the artery segment being studied. In normal conditions, the arterial pressure measured with a deflated balloon is related to systemic pressure. An invasive pressure that is too high may indicate incorrect positioning of the catheter with the tip wedged against the vessel wall or the presence of air bubbles in the system. Continuous measurement during inflation will allow identification of the moment when the micro-balloon comes into contact with the vessel walls. In fact, there will be a reduction in the phasicity of the curve and a reduction in its amplitude. The presence of additional large feeders may delay or eliminate the pressure drop.

In addition, fluoroscopic monitoring is useful for visual confirmation of correct inflation in relation to the caliber of the vessel and maintenance of the correct positioning of the microcatheter tip. The presence of air inside the micro-balloon is not an indication of malfunction or rupture of the micro-balloon, nor does it affect performance.

After inflating the micro-balloon, the flow redistribution can be verified by standard angiographies and/or CBCT by injection through the Occlusafe device. The injection parameters should set the PSI at the value allowed by the microcatheter and flows between 1 and 1.5 ml/s, ensuring—in case of CBCT acquisition—that the injection duration is at least equal to the CBCT spin duration.

It has been demonstrated that values of balloon-occluded arterial stump pressure (BOASP) ≤64 mmHg enables preferential distribution of the embolizing agent to areas of lower resistance (such as tumoral territories) [2, 3].

Matsumoto et al. in 2015 performed a study on the modification of intrahepatic pressures using a balloon microcatheter [13]. Arterial pressure measurements were performed with deflated (systemic invasive arterial pressure) and inflated balloon (during flow occlusion, BOASP) at extra-hepatic and segmental intrahepatic arteries. These measurements revealed a different pressure drop performance in hepatic segments I, IV, VIII, and V compared to segments VI, VII, II, and III. This difference can be explained by the presence of communicating arches, which are more represented in the first group of segments, potentially making the use of b-TACE less effective in them. Therefore, the measurement of pressure becomes essential when working in the central territories, especially in the perihilar ones.

Not to be forgotten is the mechanical anti-reflux action of the device when it is used in a collateral vessel (Fig. 9.2), to protect extrahepatic territories (cystic, GDA) or to exclude arterio-portal fistulas.

9.2 Embolization Endpoint

Embolization of the nodule can be performed safely after correct positioning of the microcatheter, inflation of the balloon, and assessment of the pressure drop downstream.

The embolization must be constantly monitored under fluoroscopy to obtain a correct visualization of the emulsion deposition and to check for the possible opening of collateral circles, which will be used to establish one of the endpoints of the embolization.

The endpoint of embolization is determined by several factors, which may be defined as mechanical (the perception of resistance and reflux of the microspheres), hemodynamic (reversal of flow in collaterals, visualization of intrahepatic shunts), and chemotherapy tolerant (maximum dose of drug that can be administered to the patient).

When the vascular bed of the cancer has been completely saturated, it is also possible that intrahepatic collaterals may be opened, resulting in nontarget embolization, identifying the hemodynamic endpoint embolization (Fig. 9.5). The vascular saturation of the lesion may result in a mechanical perception of increased resistance to injection and reflux of microspheres, thus defining a new endpoint of embolization.

The chemotherapy drugs recommended by EASL-EORTC guidelines include doxorubicin or cisplatin, with a doxorubicin dose of 50–75 mg/m^2 body surface area. The maximum chemotherapy dose that can be administered in a patient undergoing TACE is on average about 100 mg, representing an endpoint of the procedure (Fig. 9.6).

Tip and Tricks If an air bubble is observed in the micro-balloon, it is sufficient to turn the bal-

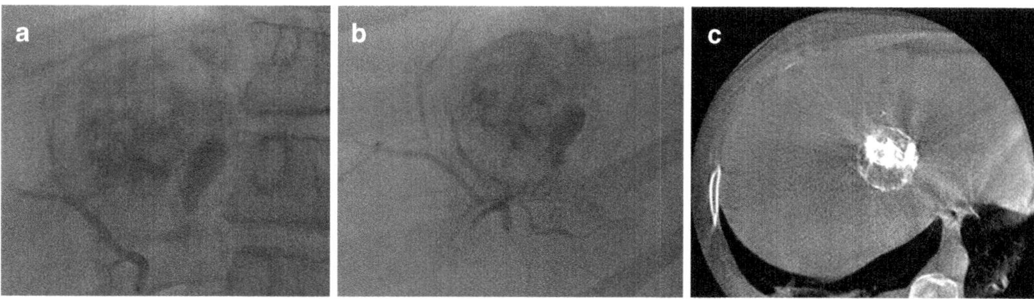

Fig. 9.5 The fluoroscopic image acquired during embolization of the HCC nodule described in Fig. 9.1 shows the "access to the microcirculation" (**a**). The endpoint of embolization was the visualization of new collateral circles not supplying the lesion due to saturation of the vascular bed of the microcirculation (**b**), obtaining complete embolization of the lesion (**c**)

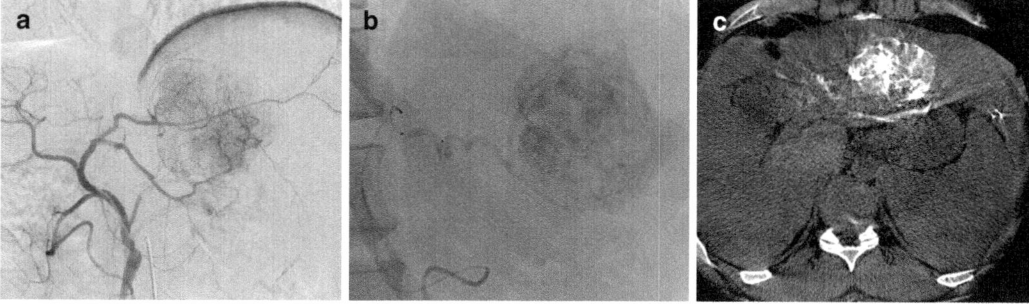

Fig. 9.6 Arteriography demonstrates an HCC of approximately 5 cm at segment II (**a**). The endpoint of embolization in this case is administration of the full dose of Farmorubicin (**b**) delivered by microparticles, showing a complete embolization of lesion and feeder artery confirmed on post-procedural cone-beam CT (**c**)

loon upside down, tap it with the finger so that the bubble is pushed to the top, and then aspirate.

References

1. Nakamura T, Oi. Hepatic embolization for the common hepatic artery using balloon occlusion technique.
2. Irie K, Takahashi. Dense accumulation of lipiodol emulsion in hepatocellular carcinoma nodule during selective balloon-occluded transarterial chemoembolization: measurement of balloon-occluded arterial stump pressure.
3. Lucatelli et al. Balloon-occluded transcatheter arterial chemoembolization (b-TACE) for hepatocellular carcinoma performed with polyethylene-glycol epirubicin-loaded drug-eluting embolics: safety and preliminary results.
4. Rose et al. The beauty and bane of pressure-directed embolotherapy: hemodynamic principles and preliminary clinical evidence.
5. Lucatelli et al. In vivo comparison of micro-balloon interventions (MBI) advantage: a retrospective cohort study of DEB-TACE versus b-TACE and of SIRT versus b-SIRT.
6. Lucatelli et al. Balloon-occluded TACE (B-TACE) vs. DEM-TACE for HCC: a single-center retrospective case control study.
7. Irie et al. Selective balloon-occluded transarterial chemoembolization for patients with one or two hepatocellular carcinoma nodules: retrospective comparison with conventional superselective TACE.
8. Golfieri et al. Balloon-occluded transarterial chemoembolization: in which size range does it perform best? A comparison of its efficacy versus conventional transarterial chemoembolization, using propensity score matching.
9. Kim et al. The safety and efficacy of balloon-occluded transcatheter arterial chemoembolization for hepatocellular carcinoma refractory to conventional transcatheter arterial chemoembolization.
10. Shirono et al. Epirubicin is more effective than miriplatin in balloon-occluded transcatheter arterial chemoembolization for hepatocellular carcinoma.
11. Hatanaka et al. Factors predicting overall response and overall survival in hepatocellular carcinoma patients undergoing balloon-occluded transcatheter arterial chemoembolization: a retrospective cohort study.
12. Matsumoto et al. Balloon-occluded transarterial chemoembolization using a 1.8-French Tip Coaxial micro-balloon catheter for hepatocellular carcinoma: technical and safety considerations.
13. Matsumoto et al. Balloon-occluded arterial stump pressure before balloon-occluded transarterial chemoembolization.

The Current Situation Regarding TACE-Specific Scores

10

Alberta Cappelli, Rita Golfieri, Violante Mulas, Antonio De Cinque, Maria Adriana Cocozza, and Cristina Mosconi

There is currently strong evidence that the optimum TACE-specific score should include tumor number, tumor size, vascular invasion, etiology, and TACE response in addition to liver function parameters, such as serum albumin and bilirubin.

These parameters have already been proposed in the hepatoma arterial embolization prognostic (HAP) score and in its modifications [1–5].

Despite the lack of validation of these scores, there is strong evidence to replace the Child-Pugh score that assesses liver function in patients with HCC with a reliable specific score capable of predicting response to treatment.

However, the "TACE population" is extremely variable and there is also wide variation in survival in the cohort classified as "ideal candidates" for TACE.

Moreover, in clinical practice, many patients receive TACE outside the guideline criteria.

Therefore, the main aim of creating a prognostic score should be to identify, on the one hand, the subgroup of patients who are *best responders* to TACE in whom retreatment is appropriate and, on the other hand, the subgroup of patients who are *worst responders* to TACE in whom other therapies may be more appropriate.

As a consequence, it is necessary to define the prognostic features and translate them into scores or "models" in order to assess prognosis at a subgroup or individual patient level as follows:

- *Scores for initial TACE.*
- *Scores for retreatment with TACE.*
- *Retreatment of refractory cases with TACE.*

10.1 Scores for Initial TACE

One of the first TACE-specific scores was the HAP score, computed using the following baseline pre-TACE scores: serum bilirubin >17 mmol/L, albumin >400 ng/mL, and tumor size >7 cm [6].

The patients were assigned one point for each of the abovementioned parameters; the HAP stages were A, B, C, and D (0, 1, 2, and >2 points) (Table 10.1).

Patients who benefited the least from TACE and had a bad prognosis were HAP stages C and D.

Park et al. [7] proposed removing the bilirubin parameter and including portal vein involvement and the modified response evaluation criteria in solid tumors (mRECIST) criteria response.

A. Cappelli (✉) · R. Golfieri · V. Mulas · M. A. Cocozza · C. Mosconi
Department of Radiology, IRCCS Azienda Ospedaliero-Universitaria di Bologna, Bologna, Italy
e-mail: alberta.cappelli@aosp.bo.it; rita.golfieri@aosp.bo.it; violante.mulas@aosp.bo.it; mariaadriana.cocozza@tudio.unibo.it; cristina.mosconi@aosp.bo.it

A. De Cinque
Interventional Neuroradiology Unit, Azienda Ospedaliero-Universitaria di Parma, Parma, Italy
e-mail: adecinque@ao.pr.it

P. Lucatelli (ed.), *Transarterial Chemoembolization (TACE)*,
https://doi.org/10.1007/978-3-031-36261-3_10

Table 10.1 Hepatoma arterial embolization prognostic (HAP) score (modified from Elshaarawy et al. 2019 [9]). Modified hepatoma arterial embolization prognostic (mHAP) II score (modified from Elshaarawy et al. 2019 [9])

	Scoring I/HAP classification	**Points**
Albumin <36 g/dL Alpha-fetoprotein (AFP) >400 ng/mL Bilirubin >17 µmol/L Max TU diameter > 7 cm	A	0
	B	1
	C	2
	D	>2
	Scoring I/mHAP II classification	**Points**
Tumor size (>7 cm) Tumor number (≥2) Alpha-fetoprotein (AFP >400 ng/mL) Bilirubin (>0.9 µmol/L) Albumin (<3.6 g/dL)	A	0
	B	1
	C	2
	D	3–5

However, additional validation of this scoring system showed no superiority when compared to the HAP score.

Nevertheless, Cappelli et al. [8] also modified the HAP score by including tumor number; the resulting score was more significant than that of the original HAP score (0.589; 95% CI: 0.552–0.626; $P = 0.001$), and the modified HAP-II score (0.611; 95% CI: 0.572–0.650; $P = 0.005$) (mHAP III). Therefore, a Web-based calculator (optimized for smartphones) was developed and published online at http://www.liver-cancer.eu/mhap3.html.

This Web-based calculator helps physicians to calculate survival in daily clinical practice.

In addition, Ogasawara et al. [9] proposed the Chiba HCC in intermediate-stage prognostic (CHIP) score (Table 10.2) that consisted of CP score plus the number of lesions and the presence of hepatitis C virus (HCV) as an etiology. However, in the end, this score was weak due to the presence of the CP score that involved a subjective assessment of encephalopathy, the number of ascites, and the predetermined cutoff points.

Table 10.2 Chiba HCC in intermediate-stage prognostic (CHIP) score (modified from Elshaarawy et al. 2019 [9]).

Prognostic factor	Points
Number of nodules	
1	0
2–7	2
8	3
CP	
5	0
6	1
7	2
8–9	3
HCV RNA positive	
Absent	0
Present	1

CP Child-Pugh, *HCV* hepatitis C virus

Op den Winkel et al. [10, 11] proposed the Munich TACE (Table 10.3) score that included alpha-fetoprotein (AFP), serum bilirubin, prothrombin concentration, creatinine, C-reactive protein (CRP), and tumor extension.

In early 2018, the authors carried out an additional validation of the proposed score and reported an area under the receiver operating characteristic (AUROC) curve of 0.71, which was superior to the TACE-tailored CLIP, HAP, Japan Integrated Staging (JIS), GETCH, BCLC, CP, Okuda, and STATE scores.

More recently, other scores, such as albumin-bilirubin (ALBI), platelet-albumin-bilirubin (PALBI), ALBI-T, modified ALBI-T, and indocyanine green retention test, showed better performance as compared to the conventional Child-Pugh score and the BCLC staging system. Campani et al. have recently compared TACE-specific scores, such as HAP, mHAP II, and mHAP III, to other general grading systems, such as ALBI and PALBI grades, on 1058 patients with intermediate-stage HCC, reporting the superiority of mHAP III over the other scores [5].

Table 10.3 Munich transarterial chemoembolization (TACE) score (modified from Elshaarawy et al. 2019 [9])

	Points				
	0	2	3	4	5
Alpha-fetoprotein (AFP) (ng/mL)	<35	–	36–999	–	≥1000
Bilirirubin (μmol/L)	<1.1	–	1.1–3.0	–	3.1
C-reactive protein (CRP) (mg/dL)	<0.5	–	0.5–1.9	–	2
Creatinine (mg/dL)	<1.3	≥1.3	–	–	–
Tumor extension	Category A[a]	–	–	Category B[b]	–
Quick (MELD)	≥75	<75	–	–	–

[a]Category A. Stage I: 0–9 points. Stage II: 10–13 points. Stage III: 14–26 points
[b]Category B: Large (one nodule >5 cm) or multilocular (exceeding the limits of 3 nodules ≤3 cm) or having vascular involvement

10.2 Scores for Retreatment with TACE

Assessment for Retreatment with TACE (ART) was the first score to list the retreatment strategies with TACE (Table 10.4). In a cohort of 107 patients with BCLC stages A and B who underwent two TACE sessions within 90 days, Sieghart et al. [12] reported two groups of patients (0–1.5 and > 2.5 points) with better survival in the first group (23.5 vs. 6.6 months; $P < 0.001$). The predictive power of the ART score for treatment response was later used by Hucke et al. [13] who proposed the STATE score and the START strategy.

The STATE score also identified two groups (<18 points, ≥18 points) with different times of survival (5.3 vs. 19.5 months, respectively, $P < 0.001$). The following validation stated that the STATE score was the best tool to determine suitability for a first TACE, and the START strategy was better in the prognostic setting than the ART score [14]. However, the authors concluded the limited ability of all these scores.

In 2015 [15], the alpha-fetoprotein, BCLC, CP, and response (ABCR) score was proposed (Table 10.5) based on baseline BCLC stage AFP level (>200 ng/mL = +1 point) in addition to pre-second TACE Child-Pugh score and radiologic tumor response. Patients with ABCR score ≥ 4 prior to the second TACE would not benefit from a second treatment. However, Kloeckner et al. [16] demonstrated the poor prognostic ability of the ART and the ABCR scores as a valid tool for assessing the clinical decision-making as regards stopping TACE cycles.

Consequently, Pinato et al. validated and compared the ART and the HAP scores, concluding that the HAP score had better prognostic power; on the other hand, the ART score better predicted TACE failure. In conclusion, it was observed that the radiologic response is considered by the ART score to be an important indicator of treatment failure with TACE [17, 18].

Table 10.4 Assessment for Retreatment with TACE (ART) score (modified from Elshaarawy et al. 2019 [9])

	Score	Stage/risk group	Points
Absence of radiologic response	1	1	0–1.5
AST increase > 25%	4	2	≥2.5
CP increase			
1 point	1,5		
≥2 points	3		

AST aspartate aminotransferase, *CP* Child-Pugh

Table 10.5 ABCR score (modified from Elshaarawy et al. 2019 [9])

Prognostic factors	**Points**
BCLC stage	
A	0
B	2
C	3
AFP	1
Prognostic factor After first transarterial chemoembolization	
CP B ≥ 2 points	2
Tumor response	−3
Stage	**Points**
1	0
2	1–3
3	≥2

BCLC Barcelona Clinic Liver Cancer, *AFP* alpha-fetoprotein, *ABCR* alfa-fetoprotein, BCLC, CP, and response

10.3 Retreatment of Refractory Cases with TACE

Before planning retreatment after a TACE failure, the potential risk and benefits in terms of survival should be taken into account. Both the ART and the ABCR scores are the prognostic scores to consider for retreatment.

It has been well established that patients with >2.5 points in the ART score have shorter survival and more adverse events after a second TACE. In the same way, patients with an ABCR score ≥ 4 have no benefit of retreatment. Therefore, these scores have been questioned and have been found to be inaccurate in the decision-making process regarding retreatment.

In order to better plan a retreatment after TACE failure, it should be taken into account that TACE has an impact on liver function. For example, it has been well demonstrated that the time to decompensation was shorter in HCC patients retreated after a TACE failure than in those who switched to sorafenib [19]. Moreover, it has been well established that OS was better in patients who had <2 unsuccessful TACE procedures than in patients who had three or more TACE sessions before sorafenib [20].

To date with the emergence of regorafenib and new systemic therapies, the balance between the risks and the benefits of retreatment with TACE should be reconsidered [21].

10.4 Standardized TACE Vs. TACE on Demand

Currently, none of the scoring systems have been validated prospectively, and the timing and the maximum number of TACE sessions is still under debate.

Therefore, the maximum number of TACE sessions to be performed should be defined by a multidisciplinary tumor board, according to the distribution of the disease (monolobar/bilobar), the response of the target lesions at first TACE, and individual tolerance to the treatment.

As a consequence, TACE should not be repeated when complete necrosis is not achieved or when there is radiological evidence of progression or liver function impairment, worsening of PS, or the appearance of PVTT or extrahepatic metastases [22–24].

Transarterial chemoembolization should be repeated when imaging documents a viable tumor/partial response (PR).

There is no real consensus regarding the frequency of TACE and the interval between two TACE sessions.

A consensus of experts has proposed *on-demand repetition* rather than a *scheduled protocol* [25].

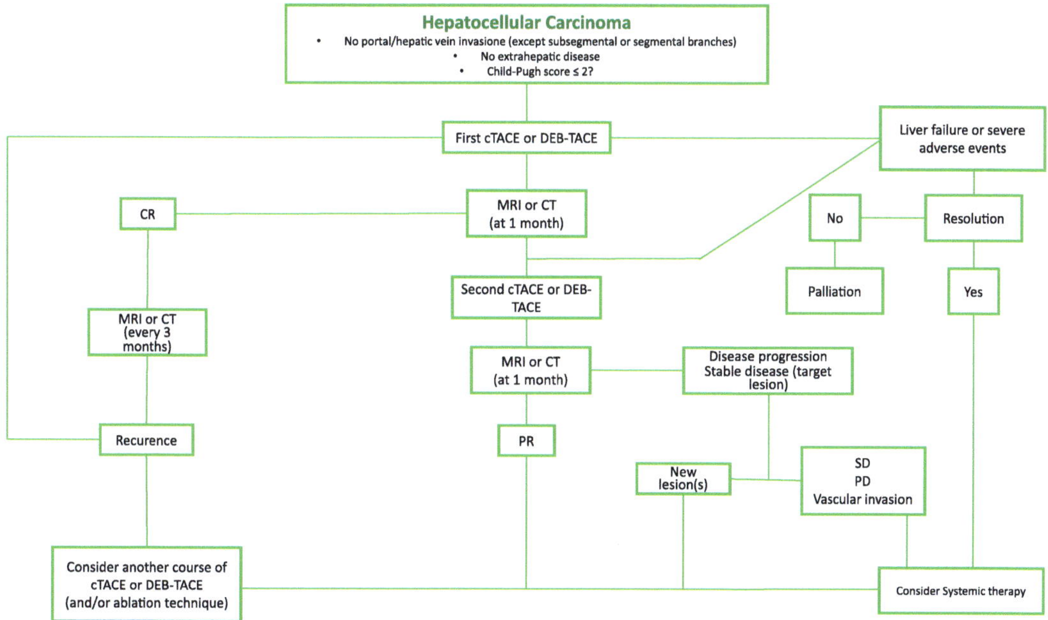

Fig. 10.1 Treatment algorithm for patients undergoing TACE (modified from Bolondi 2013 [26]). Abbreviations: *cTACE* conventional transarterial chemoembolization, *DEB-TACE* drug-eluting bead transarterial chemoembolization, *MRI* magnetic resonance imaging, *CT* computed tomography, *CR* complete response, *PR* partial response, *SD* stable disease, *PD* progressive disease

The treatment algorithm proposed by Bolondi et al. is still applied for patients undergoing TACE [26] (Fig. 10.1).

In conclusion, TACE is currently not only used for BCLC-B HCC patients; its use has been widely expanded.

Small HCCs, including hypovascular tumors, can replace surgical resection and radiofrequency ablation (RFA) in selected patients with BCLC 0-A as recently stated by the eUpdated European Society of Medical Oncology (ESMO) [27].

Moreover, in BCLC-C HCC patients with preserved hepatic function, the sequential therapy of an antiangiogenic and TACE is a promising treatment strategy [28].

However, it is important to keep in mind that TACE is not simple local chemotherapy; its outcome is strongly dependent on TACE techniques. The ultraselective procedure, with the aid of TACE guidance software, a small-sized microcatheter system and proper timing for retreatment, significantly affects the prognosis of patients having double disease, HCC, and underlying liver cirrhosis.

References

1. Waked I, Berhane S, Toyoda H, et al. Transarterial chemo-embolisation of hepatocellular carcinoma: impact of liver function and vascular invasion. Br J Cancer. 2017;116:448–54. https://doi.org/10.1038/bjc.2016.423.
2. Vincenzi B, Di Maio M, Silletta M, et al. Prognostic relevance of objective response according to EASL criteria and mRECIST criteria in hepatocellular carcinoma patients treated with loco-regional therapies: a literature-based meta-analysis. PLoS One. 2015;10:e0133488.
3. Wang W, Bai W, Wang E, et al. mRECIST response combined with sorafenib-related adverse events is superior to either criterion alone in predicting survival in HCC patients treated with TACE plus sorafenib. Int J Cancer. 2017;140:390–9.
4. Wang X, Wang Z, Wu L. Combined measurements of tumor number and size helps estimate the outcome of resection of Barcelona clinic liver cancer stage B hepatocellular carcinoma. BMC Surg. 2016;16:22.

5. Campani C, Vitale A, Dragoni G, et al. Time-varying mHAP III is the most accurate score in predicting survival in patients with hepatocellular carcinoma (HCC) undergoing trans-arterial chemoembolization (TACE). Dig Liver Dis. 2019;51:e6.
6. Kadalayil L, Benini R, Pallan L, et al. A simple prognostic scoring system for patients receiving transarterial embolisation for hepatocellular cancer. Ann Oncol. 2013;24:2565–70.
7. Park Y, Kim SU, Kim BK, et al. Addition of tumor multiplicity improves the prognostic performance of the hepatoma arterial-embolization prognostic score. Liver Int. 2016;36:100–7.
8. Cappelli A, Cucchetti A, Cabibbo G, et al. Refining prognosis after trans-arterial chemo-embolization for hepatocellular carcinoma. Liver Int. 2016;36:729–36.
9. Elshaarawy O, Gomaa A, Omar H, Rewisha E, Waked I. Intermediate stage hepatocellular carcinoma: a summary review. J Hepatocell Carcinoma. 2019;6:105–17.
10. Op Den Winkel M, Nagel D, Op Den Winkel P, et al. The Munich-transarterial chemoembolisation score holds superior prognostic capacities compared to TACE-tailored modifications of 9 established staging systems for hepatocellular carcinoma. Digestion. 2019;100(1):15–26.
11. Op Den Winkel M, Nagel D, Op Den Winkel P, et al. Transarterial chemoembolization for hepatocellular carcinoma: development and external validation of the Munich-TACE score. Eur J Gastroenterol Hepatol. 2018;30:44–53.
12. Sieghart W, Hucke F, Pinter M, et al. The ART of decision making: retreatment with transarterial chemoembolization in patients with hepatocellular carcinoma. Hepatology. 2013;57:2261–73.
13. Hucke F, Pinter M, Graziadei I, et al. How to STATE suitability and START transarterial chemoembolization in patients with intermediate stage hepatocellular carcinoma. J Hepatol. 2014;61:1287–96.
14. Mahringer-Kunz A, Kloeckner R, Pitton MB, et al. Validation of the risk prediction models STATE-score and START-strategy to guide TACE treatment in patients with hepatocellular carcinoma. Cardiovasc Intervent Radiol. 2017;40:1017–25.
15. Adhoute X, Penaranda G, Naude S, et al. Retreatment with TACE: the ABCR SCORE, an aid to the decision-making process. J Hepatol. 2015;62:855–62.
16. Kloeckner R, Pitton MB, Dueber C, et al. Validation of clinical scoring systems ART and ABCR after transarterial chemoembolization of hepatocellular carcinoma. J Vasc Interv Radiol. 2017;28:94–102.
17. Pinato DJ, Arizumi T, Allara E, et al. Validation of the hepatoma arterial embolization prognostic score in European and Asian populations and proposed modification. Clin Gastroenterol Hepatol. 2015;13:1204–8. e2
18. Pinato DJ, Arizumi T, Jang JW, et al. Combined sequential use of HAP and ART scores to predict survival outcome and treatment failure following chemoembolization in hepatocellular carcinoma: a multi-center comparative study. Oncotarget. 2016;7:44705–18.
19. Hiraoka A, Kumada T, Kudo M, et al. Hepatic function during repeated TACE procedures and prognosis after introducing sorafenib in patients with unresectable hepatocellular carcinoma: multicenter analysis. Dig Dis. 2017;35:602–10.
20. Galle PR, Tovoli F, Foerster F, Wörns MA, Cucchetti A, Bolondi L. The treatment of intermediate stage tumours beyond TACE: from surgery to systemic therapy. J Hepatol. 2017;67:173–83.
21. Kohla MAS, Abu Zeid MI, Al-Warraky M, Taha H, Gish RG. Predictors of hepatic decompensation after TACE for hepatocellular carcinoma. BMJ Open Gastroenterol. 2015;2:e000032.
22. Facciorusso A, Bhoori S, Sposito C, Mazzaferro V. Repeated transarterial chemoembolization: An overfitting effort? J Hepatol. 2015;62:1440–2.
23. Terzi E, Golfieri R, Piscaglia F, Galassi M, Dazzi A, Leoni S, et al. Response rate and clinical outcome of HCC after first and repeated cTACE performed "on demand". J Hepatol. 2012;57:1258–67.
24. Terzi E, Terenzi L, Venerandi L, Croci L, Renzulli M, Mosconi C, et al. The ART score is not effective to select patients for transarterial chemoembolization retreatment in an Italian series. Dig Dis. 2014;32:711–6.
25. Raoul JL, et al. Evolving strategies for the management of intermediate-stage hepatocellular carcinoma: available evidence and expert opinion on the use of transarterial chemoembolization. Cancer Treat Rev. 2011;37:212–20.
26. Bolondi L, et al. Position paper of the Italian Association for the Study of the Liver (AISF): the multidisciplinary clinical approach to hepatocellular carcinoma. Dig Liver Dis. 2013;45:712–23.
27. ESMO Guidelines Committee. eUpdate Hepatocellular Carcinoma Algorithm. Available online: https://www.esmo.org/guidelines/gastrointestinal-cancers/hepatocellular-carcinoma/eupdate-hepatocellular-carcinoma-algorithm (accessed on 19 June 2020).
28. Sato Y, Nishiofuku H, Yasumoto T, Nakatsuka A, Matsuo K, Kodama Y, Okubo H, Abo D, Takaki H, Inaba Y, et al. Multicenter phase II clinical trial of sorafenib with transarterial chemoembolization for advanced stage hepatocellular carcinomas (Barcelona Clinic Liver Cancer stage C): STAB study. J Vasc Interv Radiol. 2018;29:1061–7.

Drugs for TACE of HCC

11

Boris Guiu

11.1 Drug Choice

In a 2019 worldwide survey on TACE of HCC, doxorubicin appeared as the most popular drug (71.7% of responders) especially in Europe, North America, and Korea, whereas pirarubicin was the most commonly used in China and epirubicin in Japan [1]. Beyond these trends, most available chemotherapeutic agents have been or are used for HCC TACE, either alone or in combination. Of note, most of these drugs are not approved by health authorities for TACE of HCC.

11.1.1 Doxorubicin in HCC: Widely Adopted despite Outdated and Never-Reproduced Data

The first way to select the optimal drug for HCC TACE is to use a drug that has shown significant clinical efficacy through intravenous administration. If this drug has a high hepatic extraction ratio, this may be a good candidate for TACE.

Data in favor of doxorubicin in HCC come from only two (very old) studies: The first one was a single-arm phase II study conducted in 1975 [2] where 14 HCC patients were treated by IV doxorubicin. A tumor response was documented in 11/14 patients, among whom three presented complete response. Importantly, only ultrasonography was available for evaluating tumor response at that time. The second one was a case-series published in 1978 that reported 32% of clinical response after treatment by 60 mg/m^2 doxorubicin. Of note, the promising results reported in these studies from the 1970s have never been reproduced so far. Only one randomized trial showed a benefit for systemic doxorubicin (over nolatrexed) [3], whereas all the others were negative [4–6]. In a very recent randomized phase III trial, Abou-Alfa and colleagues acknowledged that doxorubicin does not have a role as a systemic therapy for patients with advanced HCC [7], in keeping with clinical results observed in HCC over the past 40 years. Nowhere is doxorubicin used as a systemic treatment for HCC.

Despite poor rationale for doxorubicin, the randomized trial published by Llovet et al. in the Lancet in 2002 [8] demonstrated that TACE (with doxorubicin) improved survival compared to best supportive care. Of note, randomization in this study was performed between three groups (TACE, best supportive care, and embolization alone). Unfortunately, the trial was stopped prematurely because TACE was proved superior to BSC, thereby preventing any comparison between TACE (with doxorubicin) and embolization. In the same year, Lo et al. [9] also reported a survival benefit with TACE but using cisplatin

B. Guiu (✉)
Department of Radiology, St-Eloi University Hospital, Montpellier, France
e-mail: b-guiu@chu-montpellier.fr

P. Lucatelli (ed.), *Transarterial Chemoembolization (TACE)*,
https://doi.org/10.1007/978-3-031-36261-3_11

(not doxorubicin). Based on these two randomized trials, TACE was recommended as the first-line treatment for BCLC B HCC patients. The widespread adoption of doxorubicin for TACE certainly came up from its good safety profile (although no phase I had ever been conducted), low cost, positive results (over BSC) in the study by Llovet et al., and promising data from initial studies despite previously mentioned strong limitations.

A randomized phase II trial (again published by the group of Abou-Alfa) published in the Journal of Clinical Oncology in 2016 has reopened the debate by showing no difference in terms of response and survival between doxorubicin-eluting bead TACE and bland embolization [10]. This led the authors to conclude that "these results challenge the use of doxorubicin-eluting beads for chemoembolization of HCC." In this study, the same embolic was injected in both arms and only the use of doxorubicin differed. The efficacy of doxorubicin was therefore seriously called into question.

In 2013, a randomized trial has been reported in 365 patients and showed that a triple-drug (lobaplatin, epirubicin, and mitomycin C) TACE regimen was associated with OS benefit compared to single-drug (epirubicin) TACE [11]. Additionally, this trial highlighted that triple-drug chemolipiodolization (i.e., transarterial injection of a chemotherapeutic agent emulsified with lipiodol without any embolizing agent) provided similar results as compared to triple-drug TACE, thereby suggesting that embolization is not mandatory to efficiently treat HCC intra-arterially. Likewise, three additional randomized trials failed to show any survival differences between chemolipiodolization and TACE in unresectable HCC patients [12–14]. Therefore, the mechanisms by which TACE improves patient survival remains to be clarified, and one should avoid any dogmatism regarding the relative contribution of the drug(s) and the embolizing agent(s) with regard to the antitumor efficacy.

11.1.2 Building the Rationale of a Drug for HCC TACE: The Example of Idarubicin

The absence of robust data on drug efficacy in HCC led to conduct a cytotoxicity study in 2011 to screen 11 drugs against three HCC cell lines [15] with the aim to select the most efficient for further clinical studies. It is well known that TACE procedure varies widely across centers and interventional radiologists, especially regarding chemotherapeutic drugs, doses, drug-releasing platforms, and embolizing agents [16, 17]. By directly testing drugs on HCC cells, the own efficacy of the drug was actually captured without any confounder. The in vitro screening study demonstrated that the anthracycline idarubicin was the most cytotoxic drug, far more than the other agents, including doxorubicin [15]. The greater cytotoxicity of idarubicin on HCC cells had two main explanations: its highly lipophilic nature resulting in an increased penetration of the drug through the lipophilic double layer of tumor cells [18, 19] and its ability to overcome the multidrug resistance system [20]—able to pump the drugs out of tumor cells—typically observed in HCC [21].

Excellent safety profile and promising clinical efficacy of idarubicin-loaded beads have been reported in phase I and II studies when using 10 mg of idarubicin [22, 23]. Due to the low lipophilicity of doxorubicin, doxorubicin-lipiodol emulsions are very unstable [19, 24], thus explaining the fast systemic diffusion of doxorubicin and the absence of pharmacokinetic (PK) advantage of doxorubicin-lipiodol over IA doxorubicin [25, 26]. Indeed, PK studies revealed no differences in terms of maximal concentration (C_{max}) of doxorubicin in plasma whether it was injected intravenously or intra-arterially, with or without lipiodol [25, 26]. By contrast, and owing to the higher lipophilicity of idarubicin vs. doxorubicin, idarubicin-lipiodol emulsion is extremely stable [19]. Therefore, idarubicin can take advantage of the tumor vectorization property of lipiodol [27] with a favorable PK profile [15, 19]. Safety profile and first data on clinical efficacy of cTACE using idarubicin were then published [28].

Based on its high cytotoxicity on HCC cells [15], high hepatic extraction ratio (40% of the injected dose distributed in the liver), and high lipophilicity leading to stable emulsions with lipiodol [19], the concept of chemolipiodolization was revisited through the conduction of the LIDA-B dose-escalation phase I [29]. It was hypothesized that idarubicin mixed with lipiodol could be administered in an "oncological" regimen, meaning every 2–3 weeks, to limit the tumor repopulation phenomenon that occurs between TACE sessions. Indeed, embolization that is basically part of TACE mandates the administration of TACE sessions every 4–8 weeks to maintain acceptable tolerance for the patient. With idarubicin, chemolipiodolization could therefore be both effective and safe as compared to TACE, given the absence of embolization [29]. The LIDA-B phase I trial reported a maximum tolerated dose of idarubicin reaching 20 mg, an objective response rate of 29%, and an encouraging survival data. The LIDA-B II multicenter phase II trial is currently ongoing in France in order to explore whether idarubicin-lipiodol can provide tumor control and keep TACE as a second-line treatment in case of tumor progression.

To sum up, strong rationale, very good safety profile, and promising clinical efficacy have been reported for idarubicin in cTACE [28], DEM-TACE [23], and chemolipiodolization [29]. However, no prospective randomized data are available so far and are very unlikely to become available in the future for at least three reasons: The first one is the high difficulty to choose a validated standard regimen, doxorubicin being the most logical but at the same time the poorest in terms of rationale; the second is the need to include ≈1000 patients to draw realistic statistical hypotheses regarding a phase III trial comparing drugs; the last relates on the large funding necessary to conduct such trial in a context where idarubicin, like doxorubicin, and most chemotherapeutic agents are genericized.

11.2 Drug Dose

The drug dose is also strongly heterogeneous among centers and radiologists. Drug dosage can be determined by a fixed dose, or based on body surface area (BSA), tumor size, body weight, or bilirubin level [1, 16]. By comparison in oncology, all chemotherapeutic agents (except carboplatin) are administered using a dosage calculated on BSA. One reason for that relies on toxicity: Cardiotoxicity of anthracyclines (doxorubicin, epirubicin, idarubicin) is cumulative and observed above a certain threshold, for example, 450 mg/m^2 for doxorubicin. It means that a typical patient of 1.6 m^2 and 60 kg has a 1.6 m^2 BSA. Four sessions of 150 mg doxorubicin TACE can be performed safely with regard to cardiac toxicity, but not more.

In oncology, the widely accepted way to determine the optimal dose is to conduct dose-escalation phase I trials. With DEM-TACE, maximum tolerated dose for idarubicin was 10 mg whereas it was 20 mg with idarubicin lipiodolization. With doxorubicin DEM-TACE, no dose-limiting toxicity was reported in a dose-escalation phase I testing 25–150 mg of doxorubicin [30], explaining why 150 mg was recommended for further trials (notably PRECISION V). Such data are not available with doxorubicin cTACE. Whatever the empiric choice of drug dose for anthracyclines, it can be recommended to keep cumulative dose below the cardiac toxicity threshold and to pay specific attention to patients who may have been treated by anthracyclines in the past (typically in breast cancer patients where epirubicin is the most frequently used anthracycline) or who present any heart disease or failure.

11.3 TACE and Systemic Drugs

11.3.1 TACE Combined with Tyrosine Kinase Inhibitors and Antiangiogenics

Owing to its embolizing effect, TACE favors the release of pro-angiogenic factors (such as VEGF) that, in turn, may cause tumor progression. Post-

TACE serum VEGF levels have been associated to both response and survival, and higher VEGF levels correlated with poorer response and survival [31]. This led to conduct several phase III RCTs to assess the benefit of adding tyrosine kinase inhibitors (TKI) with antiangiogenic effects or antiangiogenic molecules to TACE (either conventional or using drug-eluting microspheres).

Sorafenib has been validated as the first systemic treatment of HCC in 2007. Three RCTs have been conducted with sorafenib in addition to TACE: the SPACE and TACE 2 trials both compared sorafenib with DEM-TACE vs. placebo with DEM-TACE, respectively, in 307 and 313 patients (primary endpoints: time-to-progression and progression-free survival, respectively). The TACTICS trial compared TACE alone to sorafenib-TACE-sorafenib (interruption for 2 days before and after TACE) (n = 228; primary endpoint: progression-free survival). The BRISK-TA trial evaluated brivanib after TACE vs. placebo after TACE (n = 502; main endpoint: overall survival), and the ORIENTAL trial compared orantinib with TACE vs. placebo with TACE (n = 889; main endpoint: overall survival) [32]. Despite the high number of patients included in these trials, all of them were negative except the TACTICS trial [33], showing a benefit in PFS (25.2 vs. 13.5 months; $p = 0.006$).

11.3.2 TACE Combined With or Against Immune-Checkpoint Inhibitors

The combination of immunotherapy (atezolizumab) and anti-VEGF (bevacizumab) has become the new standard for the first-line treatment of advanced HCC [34]. Many RCTs involving immune-checkpoint inhibitors (ICIs) combined with TKI or antiangiogenics are ongoing in the field of HCC. By inducing tumor cell death, TACE may trigger anticancer immune response, explaining that several trials are exploring potential synergies between TACE and immunotherapies. Different associations are tested in RCTs: TACE +/− durvalumab +/− bevacizumab (EMERALD-1 trial), TACE +/− (pembrolizumab + lenvatinib) (LEAP-012), TACE +/− (atezolizumab + bevacizumab) (ML42612), and TACE +/− (nivolumab + ipilimumab) (CHECKMATE-74 W) [32].

The ≈30% objective response rate (upon mRECIST) obtained by atezolizumab + bevacizumab, as well as several other combinations of ICIs + TKI/antiangiogenics, tends to reach the objective response rate of TACE itself. This explains why two RCTs are starting not in combination with TACE but against TACE: TACE vs. atezolizumab + bevacizumab (ABC-HCC trial) and TACE vs. nivolumab + regorafenib (RENOTACE trial).

The results of all these RCTs are pending and might define new standards in the future.

References

1. Young S, Craig P, Golzarian J. Current trends in the treatment of hepatocellular carcinoma with transarterial embolization: a cross-sectional survey of techniques. Eur Radiol. 2019;29(6):3287–95.
2. Olweny CL, Toya T, Katongole-Mbidde E, Mugerwa J, Kyalwazi SK, Cohen H. Treatment of hepatocellular carcinoma with Adriamycin. Preliminary communication. Cancer. 1975;36(4):1250–7.
3. Gish RG, Porta C, Lazar L, Ruff P, Feld R, Croitoru A, et al. Phase III randomized controlled trial comparing the survival of patients with unresectable hepatocellular carcinoma treated with nolatrexed or doxorubicin. J Clin Oncol. 2007;25(21):3069–75.
4. Lai CL, Wu PC, Lok AS, Lin HJ, Ngan H, Lau JY, et al. Recombinant alpha 2 interferon is superior to doxorubicin for inoperable hepatocellular carcinoma: a prospective randomised trial. Br J Cancer. 1989;60(6):928–33.
5. Mok TS, Leung TW, Lee SD, Chao Y, Chan AT, Huang A, et al. A multi-Centre randomized phase II study of nolatrexed versus doxorubicin in treatment of Chinese patients with advanced hepatocellular carcinoma. Cancer Chemother Pharmacol. 1999;44(4):307–11.
6. Yeo W, Mok TS, Zee B, Leung TW, Lai PB, Lau WY, et al. A randomized phase III study of doxorubicin versus cisplatin/interferon alpha-2b/doxorubicin/fluorouracil (PIAF) combination chemotherapy for unresectable hepatocellular carcinoma. J Natl Cancer Inst. 2005;97(20):1532–8.
7. Abou-Alfa GK, Shi Q, Knox JJ, Kaubisch A, Niedzwiecki D, Posey J, et al. Assessment of treatment with sorafenib plus doxorubicin vs sorafenib alone in patients with advanced hepatocellular car-

cinoma: phase 3 CALGB 80802 randomized clinical trial. JAMA Oncol. 2019;5(11):1582–8.
8. Llovet JM, Real MI, Montaña X, Planas R, Coll S, Aponte J, et al. Arterial embolisation or chemoembolisation versus symptomatic treatment in patients with unresectable hepatocellular carcinoma: a randomised controlled trial. Lancet. 2002;359(9319):1734–9.
9. Lo CM, Ngan H, Tso WK, Liu CL, Lam CM, Poon RT, et al. Randomized controlled trial of transarterial lipiodol chemoembolization for unresectable hepatocellular carcinoma. Hepatology. 2002;35(5):1164–71.
10. Brown KT, Do RK, Gonen M, Covey AM, Getrajdman GI, Sofocleous CT, et al. Randomized trial of hepatic artery embolization for hepatocellular carcinoma using doxorubicin-eluting microspheres compared with embolization with microspheres alone. J Clin Oncol. 2016;34(17):2046–53.
11. Shi M, Lu LG, Fang WQ, Guo RP, Chen MS, Li Y, et al. Roles played by chemolipiodolization and embolization in chemoembolization for hepatocellular carcinoma: single-blind, randomized trial. J Natl Cancer Inst. 2013;105(1):59–68.
12. Yamasaki T, Hamabe S, Saeki I, Harima Y, Yamaguchi Y, Uchida K, et al. A novel transcatheter arterial infusion chemotherapy using iodized oil and degradable starch microspheres for hepatocellular carcinoma: a prospective randomized trial. J Gastroenterol. 2011;46(3):359–66.
13. Okusaka T, Kasugai H, Shioyama Y, Tanaka K, Kudo M, Saisho H, et al. Transarterial chemotherapy alone versus transarterial chemoembolization for hepatocellular carcinoma: a randomized phase III trial. J Hepatol. 2009;51(6):1030–6.
14. Kirchhoff TD, Rudolph KL, Layer G, Chavan A, Greten TF, Rosenthal H, et al. Chemoocclusion vs chemoperfusion for treatment of advanced hepatocellular carcinoma: a randomised trial. Eur J Surg Oncol. 2006;32(2):201–7.
15. Boulin M, Guiu S, Chauffert B, Aho S, Cercueil JP, Ghiringhelli F, et al. Screening of anticancer drugs for chemoembolization of hepatocellular carcinoma. Anti-Cancer Drugs. 2011;22(8):741–8.
16. Marelli L, Stigliano R, Triantos C, Senzolo M, Cholongitas E, Davies N, et al. Transarterial therapy for hepatocellular carcinoma: which technique is more effective? A systematic review of cohort and randomized studies. Cardiovasc Intervent Radiol. 2007;30(1):6–25.
17. Lucatelli P, Burrel M, Guiu B, de Rubeis G, van Delden O, Helmberger T. CIRSE standards of practice on hepatic transarterial chemoembolisation. Cardiovasc Intervent Radiol. 2021;44(12):1851–67.
18. Broggini M, Italia C, Colombo T, Marmonti L, Donelli MG. Activity and distribution of iv and oral 4-demethoxydaunorubicin in murine experimental tumors. Cancer Treat Rep. 1984;68(5):739–47.
19. Boulin M, Schmitt A, Delhom E, Cercueil JP, Wendremaire M, Imbs DC, et al. Improved stability of lipiodol-drug emulsion for transarterial chemoembolisation of hepatocellular carcinoma results in improved pharmacokinetic profile: proof of concept using idarubicin. Eur Radiol. 2016;26(2):601–9.
20. Roovers DJ, van Vliet M, Bloem AC, Lokhorst HM. Idarubicin overcomes P-glycoprotein-related multidrug resistance: comparison with doxorubicin and daunorubicin in human multiple myeloma cell lines. Leuk Res. 1999;23(6):539–48.
21. Vander Borght S, Komuta M, Libbrecht L, Katoonizadeh A, Aerts R, Dymarkowski S, et al. Expression of multidrug resistance-associated protein 1 in hepatocellular carcinoma is associated with a more aggressive tumour phenotype and may reflect a progenitor cell origin. Liver Int. 2008;28(10):1370–80.
22. Boulin M, Hillon P, Cercueil JP, Bonnetain F, Dabakuyo S, Minello A, et al. Idarubicin-loaded beads for chemoembolisation of hepatocellular carcinoma: results of the IDASPHERE phase I trial. Aliment Pharmacol Ther. 2014;39(11):1301–13.
23. Guiu B, Chevallier P, Assenat E, Barbier E, Merle P, Bouvier A, et al. Idarubicin-loaded beads for chemoembolization of hepatocellular carcinoma: the IDASPHERE II single-arm phase II trial. Radiology. 2019;291(3):801–8.
24. Favoulet P, Cercueil JP, Faure P, Osmak L, Isambert N, Beltramo JL, et al. Increased cytotoxicity and stability of lipiodol-pirarubicin emulsion compared to classical doxorubicin-lipiodol: potential advantage for chemoembolization of unresectable hepatocellular carcinoma. Anti-Cancer Drugs. 2001;12(10):801–6.
25. Kalayci C, Johnson PJ, Raby N, Metivier EM, Williams R. Intraarterial Adriamycin and lipiodol for inoperable hepatocellular carcinoma: a comparison with intravenous Adriamycin. J Hepatol. 1990;11(3):349–53.
26. Johnson PJ, Kalayci C, Dobbs N, Raby N, Metivier EM, Summers L, et al. Pharmacokinetics and toxicity of intraarterial Adriamycin for hepatocellular carcinoma: effect of coadministration of lipiodol. J Hepatol. 1991;13(1):120–7.
27. de Baere T, Zhang X, Aubert B, Harry G, Lagrange C, Ropers J, et al. Quantification of tumor uptake of iodized oils and emulsions of iodized oils: experimental study. Radiology. 1996;201(3):731–5.
28. Favelier S, Boulin M, Hamza S, Cercueil JP, Cherblanc V, Lepage C, et al. Lipiodol trans-arterial chemoembolization of hepatocellular carcinoma with idarubicin: first experience. Cardiovasc Intervent Radiol. 2013;36(4):1039–46.
29. Guiu B, Jouve JL, Schmitt A, Minello A, Bonnetain F, Cassinotto C, et al. Intra-arterial idarubicin_lipiodol without embolisation in hepatocellular carcinoma: the LIDA-B phase I trial. J Hepatol. 2018;68(6):1163–71.
30. Poon RT, Tso WK, Pang RW, Ng KK, Woo R, Tai KS, et al. A phase I/II trial of chemoembolization for hepatocellular carcinoma using a novel intra-arterial drug-eluting bead. Clin Gastroenterol Hepatol. 2007;5(9):1100–8.
31. Sergio A, Cristofori C, Cardin R, Pivetta G, Ragazzi R, Baldan A, et al. Transcatheter arterial chemoembolization (TACE) in hepatocellular carci-

noma (HCC): the role of angiogenesis and invasiveness. Am J Gastroenterol. 2008;103(4):914–21.
32. Llovet JM, Kelley RK, Villanueva A, Singal AG, Pikarsky E, Roayaie S, et al. Hepatocellular carcinoma. Nat Rev Dis Primers. 2021;7(1):6.
33. Kudo M, Ueshima K, Ikeda M, Torimura T, Tanabe N, Aikata H, et al. Randomised, multicentre prospective trial of transarterial chemoembolisation (TACE) plus sorafenib as compared with TACE alone in patients with hepatocellular carcinoma: TACTICS trial. Gut. 2020;69(8):1492.
34. Reig M, Forner A, Rimola J, Ferrer-Fábrega J, Burrel M, Garcia-Criado A, et al. BCLC strategy for prognosis prediction and treatment recommendation Barcelona Clinic Liver Cancer (BCLC) staging system. The 2022 update. J Hepatol. 2021;

Combined Therapy (TACE and Percutaneous Treatment)

12

Roberto Iezzi, Andrea Contegiacomo, Alessandro Tanzilli, and Alessandro Posa

Learning Objectives

- To explain the role of combined therapy in expanding the safety and efficacy of curative locoregional treatment strategies.
- To describe the variety of combined treatments, the technical aspects, and the rationale behind them in order to obtain the best curative results.
- To depict the current indications and future perspectives of combined therapy.

12.1 Introduction

The continuous research in locoregional curative therapies, designed to reduce the number of oncologic patients undergoing palliative treatments, is getting more and more results. One of the most interesting among these is the combination of percutaneous and intra-arterial treatments for primary and secondary liver neoplasms.

Both these locoregional liver therapies are well known for their advantages, but also come with some limitations when administered alone. In fact, ablative treatments achieve high complete response rates but only in cases of single (or few) neoplastic lesions under 3 cm, classified as early-stage according to the Barcelona Clinic Liver Cancer (BCLC) staging system (BCLC-A).

On the other side, treatments of choice for patients in the intermediate stage (BCLC-B) are intra-arterial therapies, performed with a super-selective or selective/lobar approach treating more lesions at a time but with a lower complete response and higher recurrence rates, substantially deeming it as palliative treatment [1–5].

In the last decade, the multimodal approach combining ablative and intra-arterial treatments has gradually proven its effectiveness in granting high complete response rates and low recurrence rates, mostly in the treatment of hepatocellular carcinoma (HCC), increasing the number of patients amenable for curative treatment, especially for those who have a large neoplastic lesion (exceeding 3 cm in size) or multifocal lesions not amenable for surgical resection, and reducing the indication to palliative therapies [6–8].

12.2 Rationale

Combination of percutaneous tumor ablation and transarterial chemoembolization (TACE) represents a promising strategy to increase the number of patients amenable for curative treatment, espe-

R. Iezzi (✉) · A. Contegiacomo · A. Tanzilli · A. Posa
Fondazione Policlinico A Gemelli - IRCCS - Università Cattolica del Sacro Cuore, Rome, Italy
e-mail: andrea.contegiacomo@policlinicogemelli.it

P. Lucatelli (ed.), *Transarterial Chemoembolization (TACE)*,
https://doi.org/10.1007/978-3-031-36261-3_12

cially for those who have a large neoplastic lesion (exceeding 3 cm in size) or multifocal lesions not amenable for surgical resection, thus reducing the indication for palliative therapies [9].

One of the greatest limitations of ablative treatments is the size of the lesion, related to low complete response rates for lesions larger than 3 cm; in addition, these treatments are not recommended for patients with multiple lesions, in which TACE is the most suitable approach [10].

The rationale behind combined therapies is to obtain an adequate tumor-free margin, increasing the volume of coagulation necrosis induced by ablative treatments by minimizing heat loss due to perilesional vessels through intra-arterial embolization procedures: TACE decreases the heat dispersion during ablation by reducing or occluding tumoral bloodstream and promoting tumor destruction by ischemic damage.

In the meantime, the thermal ablation, as well, could decrease the chemotherapy dose during TACE with less toxicity to the liver parenchyma while increasing drug delivery by inducing locoregional hyperemia. These two treatments combined can expand the treatment volume, granting better safety margins and longer progression-free survival [11, 12].

12.3 Clinical Indications

Currently, there is no guideline giving standardized indications for the use of combined treatments, both for HCC and liver metastases. Therefore, indications to this kind of treatment must be evaluated by a multidisciplinary group on a per-patient basis: Accurate multidisciplinary evaluation of every patient (assessing liver function, performance status, procedural and anesthesiological risks, patient's preference) is mandatory to provide the most accurate and personalized therapy; at the same time, tumor characteristics (size, location, surrounding structures, etc.) play an important role in treatment choice. Combined treatments can expand the indications for lesions amenable for curative therapies offering a better disease control in case of candidate patients for palliative therapies only; this statement is particularly true and has been thoroughly investigated in HCC patients.

12.3.1 HCC

Treatment selection for HCC patients is currently based on the Barcelona Clinic Liver Cancer (BCLC) staging system and, more recently, on the ITALICA (ITAlian LIver CAncer) staging system. However, the treatment selection process can be complicated by the extreme variability of patients' clinical status and tumor burden, requiring a multidisciplinary approach and stimulating the application of innovative treatments, such as combined therapies, in order to get the best treatment outcome.

The association between TACE and ablation showed improvements in the overall survival rates when compared to ablation alone, in patients with a single HCC lesion larger than 3 cm, without increasing the complications rate [13].

In addition, combined therapies proved to have good overall survival compared to surgical resection and can be considered in early HCCs when surgical resection is contraindicated or refuted [11, 14–16].

On the other hand, in intermediate-stage HCC patients, combined treatments can help obtain a better overall survival, quality of life, and treatment efficacy than TACE alone due to their complementary effect in reducing perilesional satellitosis and obtaining a better necrotic volume that can lead to a reduction in the number of treatment sessions, without affecting liver function [15, 17–19].

A great advantage of combined treatments is the opportunity to treat complex lesions and complex patients: It could make possible the complete and safe treatment of lesions in which ablation alone is not advised, such as lesions adjacent to extrahepatic structures like the diaphragm, the bowel loops, or the hilar region in which the risk of thermal damage is significant [20]; in these cases, ablation can be performed in the lesion's portion distant from these structures, whereas TACE is administered in the peripheral portion.

This approach can also help treat patients with a high risk of bleeding, as post-ablation TACE can treat ablation-induced bleeding [21–27].

12.3.2 Intrahepatic Cholangiocellular Carcinoma

Intrahepatic cholangiocarcinoma (ICC) is the second most common primary liver cancer, accounting for 5–10% of liver malignancies [28]. In the last few years, image-guided thermal ablation has been used for the treatment of advanced ICC with encouraging results [29–31].

A recent retrospective study on 36 lesions (24 patients) underlined that the combined treatment (ablation plus simultaneous TACE) for unresectable ICC had better results in terms of overall survival when compared to ablation or TACE alone. A conventional TACE (c-TACE) protocol was carried out using oxaliplatin and gemcitabine. US-guided percutaneous MWA was performed with a maximum power of 100 W for 8–10 minutes under local or general anesthesia. For tumors smaller than 3 cm, a single ablation was performed, while for lesions exceeding 3 cm, multiple ablations were done [32].

12.3.3 Liver Metastases from Colorectal Cancer (mCRC)

At the time of diagnosis, only a small percentage of patients with liver metastases are suitable for surgical resection. In this setting, locoregional treatments could represent a great help, and combined treatment's aim is to reduce the tumor burden. These treatments can achieve positive results, especially in unresectable oligometastatic liver-only tumors.

Colorectal cancer is the third cause of cancer death worldwide. Half of these patients develop liver metastases during the disease [33]. TACE is a potential adjuvant therapy for unresectable colorectal liver metastases (CRLM), delivering a high dose of chemo agents directly into the liver and causing lesions, ischemia, and necrosis [34]. Moreover, MWA and RFA have shown promising results as an alternative treatment in unresectable patients with oligometastatic disease [35].

A recent retrospective study on simultaneous combined treatment (TACE + ablation) in 30 patients with unresectable CRLM (with bilobar disease or nontechnically resectable metastases) showed promising results: The authors performed US-guided MWA with a single ablation for metastases less than 3 cm in diameter, while multiple ablations for larger lesions or for multiple metastases were performed. Post-procedural angiography was employed to evaluate the ablative results, and the treatment was completed with selective or superselective chemoembolization using a mixture of chemotherapeutic agents (oxaliplatin, epirubicin, and ethiodized oil). This study demonstrated that the combination of TACE + MWA was safe and tolerable, and could be considered as an alternative treatment option for unresectable CRLM, even though further studies are needed to establish the efficacy of the combined treatment [36].

12.3.4 Liver Metastases from Neuroendocrine Tumors (NET)

Neuroendocrine tumors (NET) are rare neoplasms that have most of the times an indolent natural history, with a better survival when compared to adenocarcinomas arising from the same organs [37].

However, neuroendocrine liver metastases can lead to incapacitating symptoms and could reduce long-term survival [38, 39]. Treatment of neuroendocrine liver metastases is an effective way to treat metastasis-related symptoms like pain, hematochezia, diarrhea, flush, jaundice, vomiting, and fever. Hepatic ablation and liver-directed intra-arterial therapies are possible alternatives to adjuvant locoregional intervention [40]. Ablation as well as transarterial chemoembolization showed to be safe and lead to significant symptom control for patients with metastatic G3 NETs [41, 42].

A retrospective study of 60 patients with NET liver metastases, published in 2005, analyzes the different outcomes of combined treatment of TACE plus surgical resection or cryoablation versus medical treatment or resection/cryoablation alone. TACE was performed using cisplatin, Adriamycin, and mitomycin C. Medical treatment involved chemotherapy and external-beam radiation or somatostatin analogs (octreotide and lanreotide). The combination of surgery, ablation, and chemoembolization of hepatic metastases resulted in better symptom control and improved survival; however, patients with liver involvement greater than 50% did not benefit from this approach [43].

12.4 Technical Aspects

12.4.1 Pre-Procedural Evaluation

Personalized planning and multidisciplinary evaluation of each patient, of his/her medical history and comorbidities, as well as of each target lesion, is mandatory to obtain the best therapeutic results.

All patients should be thoroughly investigated with a contrast-enhanced computed tomography (CT) or a magnetic resonance imaging (MRI) examination to assess the liver lesion burden (number, size, and location) and to evaluate liver vascular anatomy and pathology (arterial anatomical variants or the presence of arterial-portal fistulae or portal vein thrombosis (PVT).

Pre-procedural ultrasound (US) evaluation of the liver is mandatory, to assess correct visualization of the lesion(s) that will be subject to treatment, as well as to plan the best route for percutaneous approach (patient's decubitus, intercostal or sub-costal approach, degree of patient's inspiration); if the lesion is not correctly visible at the US examination, CT or cone-beam CT (CBCT) approaches can be used.

The assessment of liver function through laboratory tests (levels of aminotransferase, alkaline phosphatase, lactate dehydrogenase, total and direct bilirubin), as well as platelets count and coagulation parameters (prothrombin time, international normalized ratio (INR), fibrinogen), are also of great importance for the treatment planning.

12.4.1.1 Indications and Contraindications

Although there are still no official guidelines on combined treatments, their indications and contraindications intuitively go beyond the ones of ablative and intra-arterial therapies when considered alone. In particular, this kind of treatment is suitable for patients with a preserved liver function but large tumor burden (single target lesion larger than 3 cm in size or one large lesion and multiple small nodules), which are not suitable for transplant or surgical resection (due to age, anesthesiological risk, or patient's refusal).

Combined treatments have the same contraindication as TACE (patients with Child-Pugh class C or portal vein thrombosis) and ablative treatments (low platelet count, altered coagulative status); however, when dealing with patients with a high risk of bleeding, a particular combination of these treatments can be used to minimize the risk, as will be explained in the next sections.

12.4.1.2 Pre-Procedural Setup

All combined treatment procedures should be performed in an angiographic suite organized like a surgical theater, with continuous patient vital signs monitoring with pulse oximeter, heart monitor, and blood pressure cuff.

Anesthesiological assistance for pain management is mandatory, in particular during the ablation phase.

In general, the procedures can be performed safely during conscious sedation, even though authors in some centers prefer to perform them during general anesthesia.

Preoperative antibiotic administration is not mandatory but is greatly advised, particularly in patients with previous Oddi's sphincterotomy or biliary drainage [44, 45].

In case of liver metastases from neuroendocrine tumors (NET), patients should be premedicated with somatostatin analogues to reduce the metabolic upheaval induced by the embolization.

12.4.2 Techniques and Procedural Variations

The two main matters of debate when dealing with combined treatments are (1) the timing interval, which puts, in contrast, the historical sequential (two-step) approach versus the newly emerged single-step approach, and (2) the combination strategy, which juxtapose TACE before ablation versus ablation before TACE. Both these approaches and strategies have their advantages and limitations:

- *Sequential two-step approach* is based on performing TACE and ablation separately (from 1 day to even 30 days), following the idea that the liver needs to regenerate between the two treatments to avoid organ failure.
- *The single-step approach* includes performing both TACE and ablation (in whatever order) in the same procedure, usually with a time interval of a few minutes between one procedure and the other. This approach benefits from the use of US-guided ablation, which can be performed right in the angiographic suite. The main advantage of this approach is represented by the reduction of procedural time (when compared to the time needed to perform the two separate procedures of ablation and TACE) and costs, as well as granting a safe angiographic control over the ablation procedure (for assessing and treating bleeding complications promptly).
- *TACE before ablation approach* is based on the rationale of the reduction of the blood flow in the target lesion through the TACE, which can lead to less heat-sink effect and a better and larger ablation zone. The drawback can be represented by the risk of denaturation of the chemotherapeutic agent when exposed to the high ablative temperatures; in addition, prior TACE can result in altered US visualization of the target lesion due to the uptake of iodized oil or contrast media and the chemotherapeutic agent.
- *Ablation before TACE approach* consists of the rationale that, given the center of the lesion already targeted by the ablation, TACE will be more effective on the peripheral area of sublethal heating, which will be hyperemic and therefore can take on more chemotherapeutic agent, increasing the safety margin.

A step-by-step description of the single-step technique with ablation before TACE is reported below; it is worth remembering, however, that the single parts in which the following procedure is split into can be combined and timed at the operator's will and discretion, in order to obtain the best-personalized treatment for every single patient.

12.4.2.1 Single-Step Ablation Before TACE

1. Arterial access is obtained through a right common femoral artery or a radial access.
2. Selective left and right hepatic arteriograms and superselective catheterizations of the feeding vessels are performed with a coaxial technique through a microcatheter, injecting 4–8 mL of contrast agent at a flow rate of 2–3 mL/s to identify the tumoral feeding vessels. Microcatheters can be helpful to limit nontarget embolization to the surrounding normal liver parenchyma and to avoid spasms and ensure antegrade flow for safe delivery of embolic materials when injected through 1–5 mL Luer-lock syringes.
3. US-guided ablation of the target lesion is performed under conscious or deep sedation and local anesthesia; some authors prefer the use of general anesthesia. Power, duration, and number or ablation cycles depend on the technology adopted (RFA, MWA, cryoablation) and on the dimension and the histology of the lesion, according to the single vendor's ex vivo ablation charts.
4. Post-ablation superselective angiography is performed to evaluate the hypervascular area generated by the ablation electrodes and to assess the presence of bleeding.
5. Superselective TACE can be performed using an emulsion of chemotherapeutic agent and iodized oil ("conventional TACE," c-TACE), or using drug-eluting beads (DEB-TACE) preloaded with the chemotherapeutic drug.

6. The presence of extrahepatic feeders should be investigated in case of previously treated subcapsular neoplasms or cases of persistent neoplastic tissue with arterial feeding after treatment based on MDCT scan findings [46]. This examination helps avoid time-consuming catheterizations and the use of an excessive amount of contrast medium during the procedure [47]..
7. The vessels feeding the tumor must be all highlighted. A microcatheter could be used to select the branches feeding the tumor.
8. The aim of TACE is to obtain a stasis or near-stasis of the arterial flow in the feeding vessel, to increase the drug delivery in the target lesion. It is important to always assess the presence of reflux of chemotherapeutic drugs in nontarget vessels, which must be carefully avoided.
9. Post-procedural angiograms must be performed to evaluate the target lesion.

Intra- and Post-Procedural Care

Intraprocedural medications, including painkillers, antibiotic prophylaxis, intra-arterial lidocaine, corticosteroids, and proton pump inhibitors, are administered according to the physician's discretion. Some authors suggest obtaining pain control by narcotic administration via a patient-controlled analgesia pump. Antiemetic medication with the addition of promethazine and/or prochlorperazine, based on patient sensitivity, can be implemented if necessary and should be continued as long as needed. Post-procedural administration of antibiotics for 7–14 days is recommended by many authors to avoid liver colonization by enteric pathogens, particularly in patients with previous sphincterotomy and/or biliary drainage/stent [44, 48].

Imaging Follow-Up

Follow-up imaging should be conducted at 4–6 weeks after the treatment session. In case of lesions involving both hepatic lobes and requiring alternate bilobar treatment, imaging between treatment sessions may be avoided, based on the operator preference and/or the multidisciplinary decision.

Tumor response could be assessed according to EASL or Response Evaluation Criteria in Solid Tumors (RECIST) criteria using MRI or CT examinations performed at baseline and 1, 3, and 6 months after combined treatment, and annually thereafter. However, interpretation of tumor response based only on dimensions presents several limitations. For this reason, some variations in these criteria have been recently proposed (modified RECIST criteria) based on pre- and post-procedural lesion enhancement rather than its overall dimensions [49].

Signs of treatment response include Lipiodol uptake and absence of arterial-phase enhancement where it was present before c-TACE [50]. At MRI evaluation, the disappearance of arterial enhancement is the principal indicator of tumor necrosis [51]. Poor evidence regarding follow-up of hypovascular lesions is reported; however, an increase in the size of the target lesion, as well as enhancement in the portal-venous and delayed-phase imaging, has been described as evidence of residual/recurrent tumor [52, 53].

The emergence of one or more new lesions is considered evidence of progression in the overall patient response assessment regardless of the response obtained in target lesions. When a new or residual disease is detected, patients must be reevaluated in a multidisciplinary setting to reassess liver function and comorbidities and to identify the possibility of further treatment [53].

Complications of combined treatments sum up to those of every ablative or intra-arterial chemoembolization procedure. These can be divided into major and minor complications, immediate, periprocedural (occurring up to 30 days after the procedure), and long-term complications, based on their timing. Among major complications, there are liver abscess formation, biloma, nontarget embolization with acute cholecystitis, pancreatitis, or gastrointestinal ulceration, main vessel injury/dissection or pseudoaneurysm formation, spontaneous bacterial peritonitis, and tumor rupture [44, 54, 55]. Periprocedural and long-term complications are usually due to ischemic and metabolic liver impairment, such as biliary necrosis and liver failure [56].

Post-embolization syndrome (right upper quadrant pain, fever, increased white blood cell count, nausea, or vomiting) is common after TACE, particularly when dealing with colorectal liver metastasis treated with irinotecan, and—if self-limited—is usually not considered as a complication [54].

Future Perspectives/Procedural Variations

Improvements in techniques and materials can lead to future variations of the abovementioned "standard" technique of combined therapies, to obtain accurate ablation as well as precise and prompt delivery of the chemotherapeutic drug, with subsequent better treatment responses and less radiation dose both for operators and patients:

1. Cone-beam CT (CBCT) is lately emerging as a useful tool to accurately identify target lesions for TACE that are not visible at standard angiography or in the case of hypovascular lesions before TACE [57]. In addition, intraprocedural CBCT can be useful for the evaluation of treatment outcomes and the identification of possible nontarget embolization after TACE treatment [58].
2. A microcatheter with a micro-balloon on its tip can be used to distally occlude the feeding vessel, to drop the arterial stump pressure, and to grant a better embolization of the target lesion with less nontarget embolization, improved cancer nodule control, and enhanced procedural effects. Ablation can be performed with prior balloon occlusion of the feeding artery, to reduce the blood flow, limit the heat-sink effect, and increase the ablation volume [59].
3. Ablation procedures can also be performed under biplane fluoroscopy guidance or cone-beam CT guidance [49]. Fusion imaging can also be of great help in identifying hypovascular or isoechoic liver lesions, merging ultrasound images with pre-procedural CT, MRI, or PET-CT images [60, 61].
4. MRI-guided ablation represents one of the new frontiers in locoregional treatments, granting high accuracy and ablation control even for lesions that are not easily seen on US examination.
5. Intra-arterial chemoembolization can be substituted by intravenous systemic lyso-thermosensitive liposomal (LTL) chemotherapy: The circulating liposomal particles containing doxorubicin are destroyed by the RFA-induced target heating, determining a high drug concentration [62, 63].
6. Immunotherapy, represented by antibodies directed against tumoral neoantigens, is a promising treatment for advanced HCC and oligometastatic tumors; in this setting, locoregional liver treatments could improve neoantigens presentation and lead to a better immune response against the neoplasm; however, further studies are essential to confirm the effectiveness of this treatment and the best therapeutic modality [64–66].

12.5 Conclusions

Locoregional therapies are becoming increasingly helpful to treat unresectable primary and secondary liver lesions and, among these, combined treatments showed better efficacy and overall survival rates when compared to ablation or TACE alone, particularly in large lesions (greater than 3 cm), as well as in complex patients and complex lesions.

References

1. European Association for the Study of the Liver, European Organisation for Research and Treatment of Cancer. EASL-EORTC clinical practice guidelines: management of hepatocellular carcinoma. J Hepatol. 2012;56(4):908–43. https://doi.org/10.1016/j.jhep.2011.12.001. Erratum in: J Hepatol. 2012;56(6):1430
2. Lammer J, Malagari K, Vogl T, Pilleul F, Denys A, Watkinson A, Pitton M, Sergent G, Pfammatter T, Terraz S, Benhamou Y, Avajon Y, Gruenberger T, Pomoni M, Langenberger H, Schuchmann M, Dumortier J, Mueller C, Chevallier P, Lencioni R, PRECISION V Investigators. Prospective randomized study of doxorubicin-eluting-bead embolization

in the treatment of hepatocellular carcinoma: results of the PRECISION V study. Cardiovasc Intervent Radiol. 2010;33(1):41–52. https://doi.org/10.1007/s00270-009-9711-7.
3. Kagawa T, Koizumi J, Kojima S, Nagata N, Numata M, Watanabe N, Watanabe T, Mine T, Tokai RFA Study Group. Transcatheter arterial chemoembolization plus radiofrequency ablation therapy for early stage hepatocellular carcinoma: comparison with surgical resection. Cancer. 2010;116(15):3638–44. https://doi.org/10.1002/cncr.25142.
4. Sohn W, Choi MS, Cho JY, Gwak GY, Paik YH, Lee JH, Koh KC, Paik SW, Yoo BC. Role of radiofrequency ablation in patients with hepatocellular carcinoma who undergo prior transarterial chemoembolization: long-term outcomes and predictive factors. Gut Liver. 2014;8(5):543–51. https://doi.org/10.5009/gnl13356.
5. Cao JH, Zhou J, Zhang XL, Ding X, Long QY. Meta-analysis on radiofrequency ablation in combination with transarterial chemoembolization for the treatment of hepatocellular carcinoma. J Huazhong Univ Sci Technolog Med Sci. 2014;34(5):692–700. https://doi.org/10.1007/s11596-014-1338-5.
6. Tanaka M, Ando E, Simose S, Hori M, Kuraoka K, Ohno M, Yutani S, Harada K, Sata M. Radiofrequency ablation combined with transarterial chemoembolization for intermediate hepatocellular carcinoma. Hepatol Res. 2014;44(2):194–200. https://doi.org/10.1111/hepr.12100.
7. Yin X, Zhang L, Wang YH, Zhang BH, Gan YH, Ge NL, Chen Y, Li LX, Ren ZG. Transcatheter arterial chemoembolization combined with radiofrequency ablation delays tumor progression and prolongs overall survival in patients with intermediate (BCLC B) hepatocellular carcinoma. BMC Cancer. 2014;14:849. https://doi.org/10.1186/1471-2407-14-849.
8. Inchingolo R, Posa A, Mariappan M, Spiliopoulos S. Locoregional treatments for hepatocellular carcinoma: current evidence and future directions. World J Gastroenterol. 2019;25(32):4614–28. https://doi.org/10.3748/wjg.v25.i32.4614.
9. Iezzi R, Pompili M, Posa A, Coppola G, Gasbarrini A, Bonomo L. Combined locoregional treatment of patients with hepatocellular carcinoma: state of the art. World J Gastroenterol. 2016;22(6):1935–42. https://doi.org/10.3748/wjg.v22.i6.1935.
10. Peng ZW, Zhang YJ, Chen MS, Xu L, Liang HH, Lin XJ, Guo RP, Zhang YQ, Lau WY. Radiofrequency ablation with or without transcatheter arterial chemoembolization in the treatment of hepatocellular carcinoma: a prospective randomized trial. J Clin Oncol. 2013;31(4):426–32. https://doi.org/10.1200/JCO.2012.42.9936.
11. Rossi S, Garbagnati F, Lencioni R, Allgaier HP, Marchianò A, Fornari F, Quaretti P, Tolla GD, Ambrosi C, Mazzaferro V, Blum HE, Bartolozzi C. Percutaneous radio-frequency thermal ablation of nonresectable hepatocellular carcinoma after occlusion of tumor blood supply. Radiology. 2000;217(1):119–26. https://doi.org/10.1148/radiology.217.1.r00se02119.
12. Seki T, Tamai T, Nakagawa T, et al. Combination therapy with transcatheter arterial chemoembolization and percutaneous microwave coagulation therapy for hepatocellular carcinoma. Cancer. 2000;89:1245–51.
13. Lu Z, Wen F, Guo Q, Liang H, Mao X, Sun H. Radiofrequency ablation plus chemoembolization versus radiofrequency ablation alone for hepatocellular carcinoma: a meta-analysis of randomized-controlled trials. Eur J Gastroenterol Hepatol. 2013;25(2):187–94. https://doi.org/10.1097/MEG.0b013e32835a0a07.
14. Kim JW, Shin SS, Kim JK, Choi SK, Heo SH, Lim HS, Hur YH, Cho CK, Jeong YY, Kang HK. Radiofrequency ablation combined with transcatheter arterial chemoembolization for the treatment of single hepatocellular carcinoma of 2 to 5 cm in diameter: comparison with surgical resection. Korean J Radiol. 2013;14(4):626–35. https://doi.org/10.3348/kjr.2013.14.4.626.
15. Morimoto M, Numata K, Kondou M, Nozaki A, Morita S, Tanaka K. Midterm outcomes in patients with intermediate-sized hepatocellular carcinoma: a randomized controlled trial for determining the efficacy of radiofrequency ablation combined with transcatheter arterial chemoembolization. Cancer. 2010;116(23):5452–60. https://doi.org/10.1002/cncr.25314.
16. Yamakado K, Nakatsuka A, Takaki H, Yokoi H, Usui M, Sakurai H, Isaji S, Shiraki K, Fuke H, Uemoto S, Takeda K. Early-stage hepatocellular carcinoma: radiofrequency ablation combined with chemoembolization versus hepatectomy. Radiology. 2008;247(1):260–6. https://doi.org/10.1148/radiol.2471070818.
17. Liu HC, Shan EB, Zhou L, Jin H, Cui PY, Tan Y, Lu YM. Combination of percutaneous radiofrequency ablation with transarterial chemoembolization for hepatocellular carcinoma: observation of clinical effects. Chin J Cancer Res. 2014;26(4):471–7. https://doi.org/10.3978/j.issn.1000-9604.2014.08.18.
18. Zerbini A, Pilli M, Fagnoni F, Pelosi G, Pizzi MG, Schivazappa S, Laccabue D, Cavallo C, Schianchi C, Ferrari C, Missale G. Increased immunostimulatory activity conferred to antigen-presenting cells by exposure to antigen extract from hepatocellular carcinoma after radiofrequency thermal ablation. J Immunother. 2008;31(3):271–82. https://doi.org/10.1097/CJI.0b013e318160ff1c.
19. Iezzi R, Pompili M, La Torre MF, Campanale MC, Montagna M, Saviano A, Cesario V, Siciliano M, Annicchiarico E, Agnes S, Giuliante F, Grieco A, Rapaccini GL, De Gaetano AM, Gasbarrini A, Bonomo L, HepatoCATT Study Group for the Multidisciplinary Management of HCC. Radiofrequency ablation plus drug-eluting beads transcatheter arterial chemoembolization for the treatment of single large hepatocel-

lular carcinoma. Dig Liver Dis. 2015;47(3):242–8. https://doi.org/10.1016/j.dld.2014.12.007.
20. Morimoto M, Numata K, Kondo M, Moriya S, Morita S, Maeda S, Tanaka K. Radiofrequency ablation combined with transarterial chemoembolization for subcapsular hepatocellular carcinoma: a prospective cohort study. Eur J Radiol. 2013;82(3):497–503. https://doi.org/10.1016/j.ejrad.2012.09.014.
21. Wagner JS, Adson MA, Van Heerden JA, Adson MH, Ilstrup DM. The natural history of hepatic metastases from colorectal cancer. A comparison with resective treatment. Ann Surg. 1984;199(5):502–8. https://doi.org/10.1097/00000658-198405000-00002.
22. Jemal A, Siegel R, Ward E, Murray T, Xu J, Thun MJ. Cancer statistics, 2007. CA Cancer J Clin. 2007;57(1):43–66. https://doi.org/10.3322/canjclin.57.1.43.
23. Tamandl D, Herberger B, Gruenberger B, Puhalla H, Klinger M, Gruenberger T. Influence of hepatic resection margin on recurrence and survival in intrahepatic cholangiocarcinoma. Ann Surg Oncol. 2008;15(10):2787–94. https://doi.org/10.1245/s10434-008-0081-1.
24. Gusani NJ, Balaa FK, Steel JL, Geller DA, Marsh JW, Zajko AB, Carr BI, Gamblin TC. Treatment of unresectable cholangiocarcinoma with gemcitabine-based transcatheter arterial chemoembolization (TACE): a single-institution experience. J Gastrointest Surg. 2008;12(1):129–37. https://doi.org/10.1007/s11605-007-0312-y.
25. Frilling A, Modlin IM, Kidd M, Russell C, Breitenstein S, Salem R, Kwekkeboom D, Lau WY, Klersy C, Vilgrain V, Davidson B, Siegler M, Caplin M, Solcia E, Schilsky R, Working Group on Neuroendocrine Liver Metastases. Recommendations for management of patients with neuroendocrine liver metastases. Lancet Oncol. 2014;15(1):e8–21. https://doi.org/10.1016/S1470-2045(13)70362-0.
26. Frilling A, Clift AK. Therapeutic strategies for neuroendocrine liver metastases. Cancer. 2015;121(8):1172–86. https://doi.org/10.1002/cncr.28760.
27. Kunz PL, Reidy-Lagunes D, Anthony LB, Bertino EM, Brendtro K, Chan JA, Chen H, Jensen RT, Kim MK, Klimstra DS, Kulke MH, Liu EH, Metz DC, Phan AT, Sippel RS, Strosberg JR, Yao JC, North American Neuroendocrine Tumor Society. Consensus guidelines for the management and treatment of neuroendocrine tumors. Pancreas. 2013;42(4):557–77. https://doi.org/10.1097/MPA.0b013e31828e34a4.
28. Shaib Y, El-Serag HB. The epidemiology of cholangiocarcinoma. Semin Liver Dis. 2004;24(2):115–25. https://doi.org/10.1055/s-2004-828889.
29. Yu MA, Liang P, Yu XL, Cheng ZG, Han ZY, Liu FY, Yu J. Sonography-guided percutaneous microwave ablation of intrahepatic primary cholangiocarcinoma. Eur J Radiol. 2011;80(2):548–52. https://doi.org/10.1016/j.ejrad.2011.01.014.
30. Livraghi T, Meloni F, Solbiati L, Zanus G. Collaborative Italian Group using AMICA system. Complications of microwave ablation for liver tumors: results of a multicenter study. Cardiovasc Intervent Radiol. 2012;35(4):868–74. https://doi.org/10.1007/s00270-011-0241-8.
31. Butros SR, Shenoy-Bhangle A, Mueller PR, Arellano RS. Radiofrequency ablation of intrahepatic cholangiocarcinoma: feasibility, local tumor control, and long-term outcome. Clin Imaging. 2014;38(4):490–4. https://doi.org/10.1016/j.clinimag.2014.01.013.
32. Yang GW, Zhao Q, Qian S, Zhu L, Qu XD, Zhang W, Yan ZP, Cheng JM, Liu QX, Liu R, Wang JH. Percutaneous microwave ablation combined with simultaneous transarterial chemoembolization for the treatment of advanced intrahepatic cholangiocarcinoma. Onco Targets Ther. 2015;8:1245–50. https://doi.org/10.2147/OTT.S84764.
33. Adam R, De Gramont A, Figueras J, Guthrie A, Kokudo N, Kunstlinger F, Loyer E, Poston G, Rougier P, Rubbia-Brandt L, Sobrero A, Tabernero J, Teh C, Van Cutsem E, Jean-Nicolas Vauthey of the EGOSLIM (Expert Group on OncoSurgery management of LIver Metastases) group. The oncosurgery approach to managing liver metastases from colorectal cancer: a multidisciplinary international consensus. Oncologist. 2012;17(10):1225–39. https://doi.org/10.1634/theoncologist.2012-0121.
34. Huppert P, Wenzel T, Wietholtz H. Transcatheter arterial chemoembolization (TACE) of colorectal cancer liver metastases by irinotecan-eluting microspheres in a salvage patient population. Cardiovasc Intervent Radiol. 2014;37(1):154–64. https://doi.org/10.1007/s00270-013-0632-0.
35. Liu Y, Li S, Wan X, Li Y, Li B, Zhang Y, Yuan Y, Zheng Y. Efficacy and safety of thermal ablation in patients with liver metastases. Eur J Gastroenterol Hepatol. 2013;25(4):442–6. https://doi.org/10.1097/MEG.0b013e32835cb566.
36. Wu ZB, Si ZM, Qian S, Liu LX, Qu XD, Zhou B, Zhang W, Wang GZ, Liu R, Wang JH. Percutaneous microwave ablation combined with synchronous transcatheter arterial chemoembolization for the treatment of colorectal liver metastases: results from a follow-up cohort. Onco Targets Ther. 2016;9:3783–9. https://doi.org/10.2147/OTT.S105192.
37. Moertel CG. Karnofsky memorial lecture. An odyssey in the land of small tumors. J Clin Oncol. 1987;5(10):1502–22. https://doi.org/10.1200/JCO.1987.5.10.1502.
38. Sarmiento JM, Heywood G, Rubin J, Ilstrup DM, Nagorney DM, Que FG. Surgical treatment of neuroendocrine metastases to the liver: a plea for resection to increase survival. J Am Coll Surg. 2003;197(1):29–37. https://doi.org/10.1016/S1072-7515(03)00230-8.
39. Thompson GB, van Heerden JA, Grant CS, Carney JA, Ilstrup DM. Islet cell carcinomas of the pancreas: a twenty-year experience. Surgery. 1988;104(6):1011–7.
40. Shah MH, Goldner WS, Halfdanarson TR, Bergsland E, Berlin JD, Halperin D, Chan J, Kulke MH, Benson AB, Blaszkowsky LS, Eads J, Engstrom PF,

Fanta P, Giordano T, He J, Heslin MJ, Kalemkerian GP, Kandeel F, Khan SA, Kidwai WZ, Kunz PL, Kuvshinoff BW, Lieu C, Pillarisetty VG, Saltz L, Sosa JA, Strosberg JR, Sussman CA, Trikalinos NA, Uboha NA, Whisenant J, Wong T, Yao JC, Burns JL, Ogba N, Zuccarino-Catania G. NCCN Guidelines Insights: neuroendocrine and adrenal tumors, version 2.2018. J Natl Compr Cancer Netw. 2018;16(6):693–702. https://doi.org/10.6004/jnccn.2018.0056.

41. Taner T, Atwell TD, Zhang L, Oberg TN, Harmsen WS, Slettedahl SW, Kendrick ML, Nagorney DM, Que FG. Adjunctive radiofrequency ablation of metastatic neuroendocrine cancer to the liver complements surgical resection. HPB (Oxford). 2013;15(3):190–5. https://doi.org/10.1111/j.1477-2574.2012.00528.x.
42. Arrese D, McNally ME, Chokshi R, Feria-Arias E, Schmidt C, Klemanski D, Gregory G, Khabiri H, Shah M, Bloomston M. Extrahepatic disease should not preclude transarterial chemoembolization for metastatic neuroendocrine carcinoma. Ann Surg Oncol. 2013;20(4):1114–20. https://doi.org/10.1245/s10434-012-2786-4.
43. Touzios JG, Kiely JM, Pitt SC, Rilling WS, Quebbeman EJ, Wilson SD, Pitt HA. Neuroendocrine hepatic metastases: does aggressive management improve survival? Ann Surg. 2005;241(5):776–83.; discussion 783-5. https://doi.org/10.1097/01.sla.0000161981.58631.ab.
44. Ryan JM, Ryan BM, Smith TP. Antibiotic prophylaxis in interventional radiology. J Vasc Interv Radiol. 2004;15(6):547–56. https://doi.org/10.1097/01.rvi.000024942.58200.5e.
45. Kim W, Clark TW, Baum RA, Soulen MC. Risk factors for liver abscess formation after hepatic chemoembolization. J Vasc Interv Radiol. 2001;12(8):965–8. https://doi.org/10.1016/s1051-0443(07)61577-2.
46. Kim HC, Chung JW, Lee W, Jae HJ, Park JH. Recognizing extrahepatic collateral vessels that supply hepatocellular carcinoma to avoid complications of transcatheter arterial chemoembolization. Radiographics. 2005;25(Suppl 1):S25-39. https://doi.org/10.1148/rg.25si055508.
47. Kwon JW, Chung JW, Song SY, Lim HG, Myung JS, Choi YH, Park JH. Transcatheter arterial chemoembolization for hepatocellular carcinomas in patients with celiac axis occlusion. J Vasc Interv Radiol. 2002;13(7):689–94. https://doi.org/10.1016/s1051-0443(07)61845-4.
48. Geschwind JF, Kaushik S, Ramsey DE, Choti MA, Fishman EK, Kobeiter H. Influence of a new prophylactic antibiotic therapy on the incidence of liver abscesses after chemoembolization treatment of liver tumors. J Vasc Interv Radiol. 2002;13(11):1163–6. https://doi.org/10.1016/s1051-0443(07)61959-9.
49. Lencioni R, Llovet JM. Modified RECIST (mRECIST) assessment for hepatocellular carcinoma. Semin Liver Dis. 2010;30(1):52–60. https://doi.org/10.1055/s-0030-1247132.
50. Takayasu K, Arii S, Matsuo N, Yoshikawa M, Ryu M, Takasaki K, Sato M, Yamanaka N, Shimamura Y, Ohto M. Comparison of CT findings with resected specimens after chemoembolization with iodized oil for hepatocellular carcinoma. AJR Am J Roentgenol. 2000;175(3):699–704. https://doi.org/10.2214/ajr.175.3.1750699.
51. Kubota K, Hisa N, Nishikawa T, Fujiwara Y, Murata Y, Itoh S, Yoshida D, Yoshida S. Evaluation of hepatocellular carcinoma after treatment with transcatheter arterial chemoembolization: comparison of Lipiodol-CT, power Doppler sonography, and dynamic MRI. Abdom Imaging. 2001;26(2):184–90. https://doi.org/10.1007/s002610000139.
52. Chopra S, Dodd GD 3rd, Chintapalli KN, Leyendecker JR, Karahan OI, Rhim H. Tumor recurrence after radiofrequency thermal ablation of hepatic tumors: spectrum of findings on dual-phase contrast-enhanced CT. AJR Am J Roentgenol. 2001;177(2):381–7. https://doi.org/10.2214/ajr.177.2.1770381.
53. Ernst O, Sergent G, Mizrahi D, Delemazure O, Paris JC, L'Herminé C. Treatment of hepatocellular carcinoma by transcatheter arterial chemoembolization: comparison of planned periodic chemoembolization and chemoembolization based on tumor response. AJR Am J Roentgenol. 1999;172(1):59–64. https://doi.org/10.2214/ajr.172.1.9888740.
54. Brown DB, Cardella JF, Sacks D, Goldberg SN, Gervais DA, Rajan DK, Vedantham S, Miller DL, Brountzos EN, Grassi CJ, Towbin RB, SIR Standards of Practice Committee, Angle JF, Balter S, Clark TW, Cole PE, Drescher P, Freeman NJ, Georgia JD, Haskal Z, Hovsepian DM, Kilnani NM, Kundu S, Malloy PC, Martin LG, JK MG, Meranze SG, Meyers PM, Millward SF, Murphy K, Neithamer CD Jr, Omary RA, Patel NH, Roberts AC, Schwartzberg MS, Siskin GP, Smouse HR, Swan TL, Thorpe PE, Vesely TM, Wagner LK, Wiechmann BN, Bakal CW, Lewis CA, Nemcek AA Jr, Rholl KS. Quality improvement guidelines for transhepatic arterial chemoembolization, embolization, and chemotherapeutic infusion for hepatic malignancy. J Vasc Interv Radiol. 2009;20(7 Suppl):S219–26., S226.e1-10. https://doi.org/10.1016/j.jvir.2009.04.033.
55. Sueyoshi E, Hayashida T, Sakamoto I, Uetani M. Vascular complications of hepatic artery after transcatheter arterial chemoembolization in patients with hepatocellular carcinoma. AJR Am J Roentgenol. 2010;195(1):245–51. https://doi.org/10.2214/AJR.08.2301.
56. Chan AO, Yuen MF, Hui CK, Tso WK, Lai CL. A prospective study regarding the complications of transcatheter intraarterial lipiodol chemoembolization in patients with hepatocellular carcinoma. Cancer. 2002;94(6):1747–52. https://doi.org/10.1002/cncr.10407.
57. Miyayama S, Yamashiro M, Okuda M, Yoshie Y, Sugimori N, Igarashi S, Nakashima Y, Matsui O. Usefulness of cone-beam computed tomography during ultraselective transcatheter arterial chemoembolization for small hepatocellular carcinomas that cannot be demonstrated on angiography. Cardiovasc

Intervent Radiol. 2009;32(2):255–64. https://doi.org/10.1007/s00270-008-9468-4.
58. Lucatelli P, Argirò R, Bascetta S, Saba L, Catalano C, Bezzi M, Levi Sandri GB. Single injection dual phase CBCT technique ameliorates results of trans-arterial chemoembolization for hepatocellular cancer. Transl Gastroenterol Hepatol. 2017;2:83. https://doi.org/10.21037/tgh.2017.10.03.
59. Iezzi R, Posa A, Tanzilli A, Carchesio F, Pompili M, Manfredi R. Balloon-occluded MWA (b-MWA) followed by balloon-occluded TACE (b-TACE): technical note on a new combined single-step therapy for single large HCC. Cardiovasc Intervent Radiol. 2020;43(11):1702–7. https://doi.org/10.1007/s00270-020-02583-6.
60. Oliveri RS, Wetterslev J, Gluud C. Transarterial (chemo)embolisation for unresectable hepatocellular carcinoma. Cochrane Database Syst Rev. 2011;3:CD004787. https://doi.org/10.1002/14651858.CD004787.pub2.
61. Ray CE Jr, Haskal ZJ, Geschwind JF, Funaki BS. The use of transarterial chemoembolization in the treatment of unresectable hepatocellular carcinoma: a response to the Cochrane collaboration review of 2011. J Vasc Interv Radiol. 2011;22(12):1693–6. https://doi.org/10.1016/j.jvir.2011.09.014.
62. Zamboni WC. Concept and clinical evaluation of carrier-mediated anticancer agents. Oncologist. 2008;13(3):248–60. https://doi.org/10.1634/theoncologist.2007-0180.
63. Kong G, Anyarambhatla G, Petros WP, Braun RD, Colvin OM, Needham D, Dewhirst MW. Efficacy of liposomes and hyperthermia in a human tumor xenograft model: importance of triggered drug release. Cancer Res. 2000;60(24):6950–7.
64. Singh P, Toom S, Avula A, Kumar V, Rahma OE. The immune modulation effect of Locoregional therapies and its potential synergy with immunotherapy in hepatocellular carcinoma. J Hepatocell Carcinoma. 2020;7:11–7. https://doi.org/10.2147/JHC.S187121.
65. Viveiros P, Riaz A, Lewandowski RJ, Mahalingam D. Current state of liver-directed therapies and combinatory approaches with systemic therapy in hepatocellular carcinoma (HCC). Cancers (Basel). 2019;11(8):1085. https://doi.org/10.3390/cancers11081085.
66. Shi L, Wang J, Ding N, Zhang Y, Zhu Y, Dong S, Wang X, Peng C, Zhou C, Zhou L, Li X, Shi H, Wu W, Long X, Wu C, Liao W. Inflammation induced by incomplete radiofrequency ablation accelerates tumor progression and hinders PD-1 immunotherapy. Nat Commun. 2019;10(1):5421. https://doi.org/10.1038/s41467-019-13204-3.

New Frontiers in Transarterial Chemoembolization: Combination with Systemic Therapies

13

Rafael Duran, Thierry de Baere, and Lambros Tselikas

Abbreviations

AFP	Alpha-fetoprotein
CTLA-4	Cytotoxic T lymphocyte-associated protein 4
HAIAT	Hypoxia-activated intra-arterial therapy
HAL	Hepatic arterial ligation
HAPs	Hypoxia-activated prodrugs
HCC	Hepatocellular carcinoma
HIF-1α	Hypoxia-inducible factor-1α
HMGB1	High-mobility group box 1
PD-1	Programmed cell death 1 receptor
PD-L1	Programmed cell death 1 ligand
PFS	Progression-free survival
RAGE	Receptor of advanced glycation end products
TAAs	Tumor-associated antigens
TACE	Transarterial chemoembolization
Th17	Type 17 helper T cells
Tregs	Regulatory T cells
TTP	Time to progression
VEGF	Vascular endothelial growth factor

Learning Objectives

- To understand the mechanistic advantages and rationale of TACE to be combined with systemic therapies.
- To understand how TACE-induced hypoxia may lead to detrimental effects.
- To learn the potential immunogenic effects of TACE.
- To learn new combinatorial approaches of TACE with systemic therapies.

13.1 Introduction

Transarterial chemoembolization (TACE) is commonly used to treat patients with liver cancer, in particular hepatocellular carcinoma (HCC) [1–4]. TACE achieves cancer cell death as a result of combined locoregional delivery of high doses

R. Duran (✉)
Department of Radiology and Interventional Radiology, Lausanne University Hospital and University of Lausanne, Lausanne, Switzerland
e-mail: rafael.duran@chuv.ch

T. de Baere
Département d'Anesthésie, Chirurgie et Interventionnel (DACI), Gustave Roussy, Villejuif, France

Gustave Roussy Cancer Campus, Université Paris Saclay, Saint-Aubin, France

L. Tselikas
Département d'Anesthésie, Chirurgie et Interventionnel (DACI), Gustave Roussy, Villejuif, France

Laboratoire de Recherche Translationnelle en Immunothérapie (LRTI), INSERM U1015, Gustave Roussy, Villejuif, France

P. Lucatelli (ed.), *Transarterial Chemoembolization (TACE)*,
https://doi.org/10.1007/978-3-031-36261-3_13

of chemotherapy and tumor ischemia. The standard treatment consists of cytotoxic drugs such as doxorubicin, idarubicin, or cisplatin, although no molecule has clearly demonstrated to be superior to another. Consequently, there is no standardized and widely accepted treatment regimen, although doxorubicin is the most frequently administered agent [5, 6]. TACE achieves higher drug concentration to tumors than systemic chemotherapy with significantly reduced systemic toxicity [7]. The embolization is a crucial component of TACE that prevents the washout of the administered payload, and induces tumor death and improves survival [8].

Despite technical improvements and advances in imaging guidance and tumor targeting, long-term survival of patients treated with TACE remains suboptimal, mainly due to residual/recurrent tumor [9, 10]. One of the strategies to improve patients' outcomes is to combine TACE with systemic therapies. Here we review the rationale for this combination treatment and provide an overview of clinical achievements in the field with a particular focus on patients with HCC.

13.2 Rationale for Combination Therapies

13.2.1 TACE, Tumor Hypoxia and Angiogenesis

The main anticancer effect of TACE is achieved by the embolization that generates acute tissue hypoxia at the targeted area. This TACE-induced acute hypoxia may occur in the setting of chronic tumor hypoxia, due to the poorly organized and uncontrolled cancer cell proliferation that surpasses the tumor blood, and therefore oxygen supply. If prolonged enough, TACE-induced hypoxia induces tumoral (and peritumoral) cell death. However, this low-oxygen state generates a variety of genetic and adaptive biological responses that ultimately will allow residual cancer cells not only to survive but to do so oftentimes with a more aggressive cancer phenotype [11].

Among incriminated molecular events, hypoxia-inducible factor-1α (HIF-1α) plays a central role. Under hypoxic conditions, HIF-1α accumulates and induces the expression of numerous hypoxia-response genes [12]. One of the key molecules is vascular endothelial growth factor (VEGF) whose transcription is highly activated by HIF-1α. VEGF is a key proangiogenic growth factor that has been linked to tumor growth and proliferation. Pretreatment serum VEGF levels and increased circulating levels of VEGF following TACE demonstrated to correlate with tumor burden, poor treatment response, and patient survival [13–15]. TACE-increased VEGF expression was also observed at the tissue level in the residual surviving cancer cells [16]. In fact, complex and dynamic changes of multiple proangiogenic factors happen following embolization-related hypoxia [17]. This provided the rationale to develop TACE with drug-eluting beads loaded with antiangiogenic drugs such as sunitinib and vandetanib with good anticancer efficacy in preclinical models of liver cancer [18, 19]. A pilot study using vandetanib-eluting radiopaque beads in patients with liver cancer has completed its recruitment and results are expected soon (NCT03291379).

Thus, targeting molecular pathways of hypoxia and angiogenesis has been the focus of intense research. As a result, several drugs with antiangiogenic activity and hypoxia-targeted therapies have been developed [20, 21].

13.2.2 TACE and Immune Response

TACE has the advantage (over surgery) to achieve tumor cell death in situ and targeted tumor could be used as an antigen reservoir. Thus, TACE may uncover tumor antigens that were previously hidden to the immune system allowing to generate antigen-specific T-cell responses. It is well established that the type of cell death or cell injury has an impact on subsequent immune responses. Tumor necrosis generates immunogenic responses, although some contradicting studies suggest that apoptosis triggers strong antitumor immune responses [22–24]. Among drugs used in TACE, anthracyclines, such as doxorubicin (but not cisplatin), can generate effective antitumor immune responses and thus promote immunogenic cell death [25, 26].

Preliminary data showed that TACE is able to generate inflammatory and immune responses, induce systemic cytokine level changes, and influence the T-cell repertoire.

Complex changes in systemic cytokine levels were observed early following TACE in HCC patients, suggesting that the production of these molecules by cancer cells and the immune system may be influenced after therapy [27]. Moreover, the serum levels of high-mobility group box 1 (HMGB1), receptor of advanced glycation end products (RAGE) and DNase activity, which are known immunogenic cell death markers, were impacted early after TACE in HCC patients. In particular, RAGE levels were found to be predictive of therapy response [28]. TACE demonstrated the ability to unmask tumor-associated antigens such as alpha-fetoprotein (AFP) and elicit AFP-specific CD4+ T-cell responses [29]. Similarly, specific T-cell responses to glypican-3, a cell-surface glycoprotein overexpressed in HCC tissues, were found in 44% of HCC patients treated with TACE [30]. Furthermore, the detection of tumor-associated antigens (TAAs) by CD8+ cytotoxic T cells was increased following TACE when compared to treatment-naïve HCC patients [31]. Also, HCC patients treated with transarterial embolization showed an increased frequency of TAA-specific T cells following therapy. Importantly, novel recognition of TAAs by T cells was observed in some of these patients while these peptides were not recognized before treatment. Taken together, these results demonstrated the potential of locoregional therapies to generate and enhance tumor-specific T-cell responses. When applying immune checkpoint inhibitors, a significant increase in the number of TAA-specific T cells was observed, together with an enhanced production of cytokines, suggesting that a combination with immunotherapy may be beneficial [32]. Importantly, TACE proved to decrease regulatory T cells (Tregs), which demonstrated to favor an immunosuppressive tumor microenvironment by suppressing effector T-cell responses leading to HCC progression and poor outcomes [33, 34]. In another work, type 17 helper T cells (Th17), which have important pro-inflammatory properties and play a role in autoimmunity, were significantly increased following TACE in HCC patients. Interestingly, this increased frequency of circulating Th17 cells measured after TACE was predictive of longer time to progression (TTP) and improved patient survival [35].

Although preliminary, data gathered from these early reports justify the increasing enthusiasm to combine TACE with immunotherapy.

13.3 TACE Combined with Antiangiogenic Drugs

No systemic therapy proved to be beneficial in HCC patients with advanced disease until the late 2000s, with sorafenib, an oral multi-TKI with activity against VEGF receptor, platelet-derived growth factor receptor, and Raf kinases, demonstrating a survival advantage over best supportive care [36, 37]. Recently, the combination of atezolizumab and bevacizumab was compared to sorafenib and proved to be beneficial, in particular, in terms of overall survival, and became the new first-line standard of care in the advanced-stage disease [38].

The positive results achieved in HCC patients by systemic antiangiogenic therapy led to investigate TACE in combination with these drugs, mainly sorafenib. The combination of TACE and sorafenib, either sequentially or concomitantly, demonstrated to be safe based on a large observational registry (GIDEON trial) [39, 40]. Outcomes of TACE plus sorafenib vs. TACE alone were analyzed in recent meta-analysis including 14 studies with 1670 HCC patients [41]. The combination of TACE plus sorafenib demonstrated significantly more objective response rate (RR = 1.62, 95% confidence interval (CI) = 1.34–1.94, $p < 0.00001$), disease control rate (RR = 1.43, 95% CI = 1.26–1.62, $p < 0.00001$), and 1-year overall survival (OR = 1.88, 95% CI =1.39–2.53, $p < 0.0001$). However, this improved efficacy was at the cost of an increased incidence of adverse events attributed to sorafenib for the combination group when compared to TACE alone. In contrast, other meta-analyses showed that TACE plus sorafenib may improve the TTP but failed to show any significant increase in overall survival [42, 43], although outcomes may vary across different regions and patient populations, in particular in the Asia Pacific region when compared to Western countries [43–45]. Similarly, the BRISK-TA phase III study showed that the overall survival of HCC patients treated with TACE followed by brivanib (a selective dual inhibitor of VEGF and fibroblast growth factor receptor tyrosine kinases) or placebo did not improve significantly (26.4 and 26.1 months, HR 0.90 [95% CI 0.66–1.23]; $p = 0.528$, respectively). However, median TTP was longer in the brivanib group when compared to the placebo group (8.4 and 4.9 months, HR 0.61 [95% CI 0.48–0.77]; $p < 0.0001$, respectively) [46]. Comparably, the addition of orantinib (multiple receptor tyrosine kinase inhibitor of VEGF receptor-2 and platelet-derived growth factor receptor-β) to TACE was not superior to placebo in terms of overall survival, although the TTP was significantly longer [47]. In addition, bevacizumab, a monoclonal antibody targeting VEGF, did not show any meaningful anticancer effects over placebo as adjuvant therapy of TACE [48].

In the advanced-stage HCC setting, a recent randomized controlled phase III trial compared sorafenib vs. sorafenib combined with TACE on demand. Sorafenib was administered within 3 days and TACE within 7–21 days of randomization. Although the combination therapy achieved significantly better response rate, TTP, and progression-free survival (PFS) over sorafenib, the median overall survival—study primary endpoint—was not improved (12.8 vs. 10.8 months (hazard ratio [HR] 0.91; 90% CI 0.69–1.21; $p = 0.290$, combination therapy vs. sorafenib, respectively). Of note, in a subgroup analysis, patients who were treated with at least two TACEs had a significantly better survival when compared to patients receiving sorafenib alone (18.6 vs. 10.8 months; HR 0.58; 95% CI 0.40–0.82; $p = 0.006$, respectively) [49].

Taken together, these results show that the combination of TACE and a systemic antiangiogenic drug has an anticancer effect but failed to improve survival. Many factors can influence the fact that the observed delay in tumor progression was not translated into a survival benefit for the patients. The timing (e.g., before vs. after TACE, concomitantly, sequentially), dose, duration and toxicity of antiangiogenic therapy, management of antiangiogenic therapy-related adverse effects, number of TACE sessions, and on-demand vs. scheduled TACE may explain the absence of improved survival for the combination approach. Trials with more refined designs and new and less toxic antiangiogenic molecules should be explored in future studies in combination with TACE.

13.4 TACE Combined with Systemic Immunotherapy

Immune checkpoint inhibitors have become some of the most widely prescribed anticancer therapies. Among them, cytotoxic T lymphocyte-associated protein 4 (CTLA-4) (e.g., tremelimumab, ipilimumab), programmed cell death-1 receptor (PD-1) (e.g., nivvolumab, pembrolizumab), and programmed cell death-1 ligand (PD-L1) (e.g., atezolizumab, durvalumab) are the most widely investigated drugs [50], with promising outcomes in monotherapy and combinations. Very recently, the combination of durvalumab and tremelimumab (HIMALAYA phase I/II trial) demonstrated better survival outcomes (median overall survival, 18.7 months; 95%CI, 10.8–27.3) than what has been published for sorafenib in first line [51]. These results are now being evaluated in the phase III HIMALAYA trial (NCT03298451) in which durvalumab and tremelimumab are compared to sorafenib in advanced-stage HCC patients.

The first reported feasibility and safety study combining local therapy with immune checkpoints combined tremelimumab with either percutaneous ablation (radiofrequency or cryoablation) or TACE with drug-eluting beads (DEB-TACE). Patients with HCC were administered tremelimumab every 4 weeks for 6 doses, followed by 3-monthly infusions. On day 36, patients underwent incomplete ablation or DEB-TACE. Incomplete treatments were performed to hypothetically promote inflammation and anticancer immune response, although this concept has been recently challenged [52]. Patients treated with DEB-TACE had intermediate-stage disease. No dose-limiting toxicities were observed. Most common clinical toxicities were pruritus and aminotransferases elevation. The median TTP was 7.4 months (95% CI: 2.2–19.4 months) and OS was 13.6 months (95% CI: 7.5 months, undefined) in these heavily pretreated patients. Very interestingly, objective tumor responses were seen outside of the ablated tumors or embolized area in 26% of patients [53].

An ongoing phase Ib study is investigating the safety of TACE followed by pembrolizumab. Preliminary results showed that the combination had a tolerable safety profile with no evidence of synergistic toxicity (NCT03397654) [54]. Other ongoing trials are summarized in Table 13.1.

Table 13.1 Clinical trials combining TACE and immune checkpoint inhibitors

Drug	Trial ID	Country/city	Title
Nivolumab	NCT04268888	UK	Nivolumab in Combination With TACE/TAE for Patients With Intermediate-Stage HCC (TACE-3)
Nivolumab	NCT03572582	Germany	TACE in Combination With Nivolumab Performed for Intermediate-Stage HCC (IMMUTACE)
Nivolumab	NCT03143270	USA	A Study to Test the Safety and Feasibility of Nivolumab With DEB-TACE in Patients With Liver Cancer
Nivolumab	NCT03143270	USA	A Study to Test the Safety and Feasibility of Nivolumab With Drug-Eluting Bead Transarterial Chemoembolization in Patients With Liver Cancer
Durvalumab Tremelimumab	NCT0452254	Germany	Durvalumab (MEDI4736) and Tremelimumab in Combination With Either Y-90 SIRT or TACE for Intermediate-Stage HCC with Pick-the-Winner Design
Durvalumab Tremelimumab	NCT03638141	USA	CTLA-4/PD-L1 Blockade Following TACE in Patients with Intermediate Stage of HCC Using Durvalumab and Tremelimumab
Durvalumab Tremelimumab	NCT02821754	USA	A Pilot Study of Combined Immune Checkpoint Inhibition in Combination with Ablative Therapies in Subjects with Hepatocellular Carcinoma (HCC) or Biliary Tract Carcinomas (BTC)
Durvalumab Tremelimumab	NCT04988945	Hong Kong	TACE and SBRT Followed by Double Immunotherapy for Downstaging Hepatocellular Carcinoma
Pembrolizumab	NCT03397654	UK	Study of Pembrolizumab Following TACE in Primary Liver Carcinoma (PETAL)
Sintilimab	NCT04220944	China	Combined Locoregional Treatment with Immunotherapy for Unresectable HCC
Sintilimab	NCT04653389	China	Perioperative Therapy for Hepatocellular Carcinoma
Sintilimab	NCT04174781	China	Neoadjuvant Therapy for Hepatocellular Carcinoma
Tislelizumab	NCT04981665	China	A Study to Evaluate TACE Sequential Tislelizumab as Adjuvant Therapy in Participants with HCC at High Risk of Recurrence After Curative Resection
PD-1 monoclonal antibody	NCT04518852	China	TACE, Sorafenib, and PD-1 Monoclonal Antibody in the Treatment of HCC
PD-1 antibody	NCT03914352	China	A Novel Immunotherapy PD-1 Antibody to Suppress Recurrence of HCC Combined with PVTT After Hepatic Resection
Checkpoint inhibitor	NCT03817736	Hong Kong	Sequential TACE and SBT with Immunotherapy for Downstaging HCC for Hepatectomy
Checkpoint inhibitors	NCT04975932	China	Efficacy and Safety of TACE in Combination with ICIs for HCC: A Real-World Study (CHANCE001)

13.5 TACE Combined with Antiangiogenic Drugs and Immunotherapy

Among many studies reported in Table 13.2, a large randomized, double-blind, placebo-controlled, multicenter global phase III study is investigating the safety and efficacy of TACE combined with either durvalumab (arm A) or with durvalumab plus bevacizumab (arm B) compared to TACE alone (arm C) in HCC patients not amenable to curative therapy (EMERALD-1 study, NCT03778957). Six hundred patients will be randomized 1:1:1. Durvalumab is administered at least 1 week following the initial TACE, whereas durvalumab ± bevacizumab is given after at least 2 weeks following the last TACE. The primary endpoint is the PFS of arms A vs. C, and secondary outcomes are the OS, PFS of arms B vs. C, quality of life, and safety. Other ongoing trials are summarized in Table 13.2.

Table 13.2 Clinical trials combining TACE, immune checkpoint inhibitors, and antiangiogenic drugs

Drug	Trial ID	Country/city	Title
Durvalumab Bevacizumab	NCT03778957	Global	A Global Study to Evaluate Transarterial Chemoembolization (TACE) in Combination with Durvalumab and Bevacizumab Therapy in Patients with Locoregional Hepatocellular Carcinoma (EMERALD-1)
Durvalumab Bevacizumab	NCT03937830	USA	Combined Treatment of Durvalumab, Bevacizumab, and TACE in Subjects with HCC or Biliary Tract Carcinoma
Sintilimab Carrelizumab	NCT04997850	China	The Safety and Efficacy of Transarterial Chemoembolization (TACE) + Lenvatinib + Programmed Cell Death Protein 1 (PD-1) Antibody of Advanced Unresectable Hepatocellular Carcinoma
PD-1 monoclonal antibody Lenvatinib	NCT04273100	China	PD-1 Monoclonal Antibody, Lenvatinib, and TACE in the Treatment of HCC
Camrelizumab Apatinib	NCT04521153	China	Camrelizumab Combined with Apatinib Mesylate for Perioperative Treatment of Resectable Hepatocellular Carcinoma
Sintilimab Bevacizumab	NCT04796025	China	TACE Combined with Sintilimab Plus Bevacizumab Biosimilar in Hepatocellular Carcinoma (BCLC-C stage): A Prospective Single-Arm Phase II Clinical Study (T-Double)
PD-1 Inhibitor Lenvatinib Sorafenib	NCT04229355	China	DEB-TACE Plus Lenvatinib or Sorafenib or PD-1 Inhibitor for Unresectable Hepatocellular Carcinoma

13.6 Local Administration of Immunotherapies—Toward Immunoembolization

Local administration of immunotherapies is a very promising approach as it allows high intratumoral drug concentration and an improved bioavailability of the drug. At least in theory, this could diminish the on-target/off-tumor effects while keeping efficacy high [55, 56]. Interventional radiology developments make it possible to reach almost any target by either using percutaneous, intracavitary, or intravascular route [57]. Liver tumors are targets of choice as both percutaneous and intra-arterial supply are technically feasible. Moreover, the presence of liver metastases decreases the efficacy of systemic immunotherapies. The mechanism remains unclear, but immunosuppressive hepatic macrophages seem to play a key role, inducing CD8+ T cell siphoning and reduced T-cell population, diversity, and function [58].

Previous generations of immunotherapies (nonimmune checkpoint blockers), such as GM-CSF, have been emulsified with Lipiodol® in order to perform immunoembolization for liver metastases. This technique has proven to be feasible, and safe in patients with liver metastases from uveal melanomas [59], with results comparing favorably to TACE [60] or bland embolization [61]. Results of ongoing trials of intra-arterial infusion of anti-CTLA4 antibodies in advanced HCC patients are awaited (NCT04823403).

13.7 Hypoxia-Activated Prodrugs

Targeting hypoxia is a challenge in anticancer therapy. As a result, many strategies have been tested such as hypoxia-activated prodrugs (HAPs), hypoxia-selective gene therapy, and HIF-1α targeting [62]. Among these options, HAPs appear distinctly promising in combination with TACE. TACE has many mechanistic advantages in this context. High drug doses can be delivered locoregionally that may reach hypoxic niches of solid tumors, where cancer cells propagate untouched in pharmacological sanctuaries. In addition, the embolization performed in the setting of TACE provides an ideal terrain for the local targeted activation of bioreductive prodrugs. Indeed, HAPs are delivered as nontoxic prodrugs that undergo biotransformation under low oxygen concentrations to achieve cytotoxic activation. Evofosfamide is the HAP that is the most advanced in the clinic [63].

The addition of HAPs such as evofosfamide to TACE, called hepatic hypoxia-activated intraarterial therapy (HAIAT), was investigated in the rabbit VX2 model of liver cancer. The combination of TACE and evofosfamide given intra-arterially achieved smaller tumor volumes, higher necrotic fractions, and lower tumor growth rates when compared to TACE, with limited additional toxicity. A correlation was found between the degree of hypoxia and tumor necrosis establishing the *in vivo* proof-of-concept of selective HAIAT for liver cancer [64]. Another approach is to combine TACE to systemic HAPs. Hepatitis B virus X protein transgenic mice bearing HCC were injected with IV saline, doxorubicin, or tirapazamine, a HAP, followed by transient left hepatic arterial ligation (HAL) to mimic the embolization. Controls treated with saline did not show detectable tumor necrosis, only 5% of necrosis was observed in tumors treated with IV doxorubicin followed by HAL, whereas almost complete tumor necrosis was observed in animals treated with IV tirapazamine followed by HAL, demonstrating the potential of locoregional embolization combined with systemic hypoxia-activated therapy [65].

This approach was recently translated to the clinic in a phase I multicenter study done in unresectable HCC patients with preserved liver function. Two regimens were investigated: IV or intra-arterial tirapazamine followed by superselective transarterial embolization with ethiodized oil (Lipiodol) and Gelfoam slurry. Treatment was safe and tolerable. Grade ≥ 3 adverse events were hypertension and transient elevation of liver enzymes in 70% of patients, but no serious adverse event was considered drug related [66].

Other clinical studies are investigating HAPs in the setting of TACE and HCC patients are ongoing such as a phase I dose escalation study investigating the administration of evofosfamide with doxorubicin via TACE (NCT01721941), a randomized study comparing transarterial tirapazamine embolization vs. TACE (NCT03145558), and phase II study of transarterial tirapazamine embolization of liver cancers followed by either nivolumab or pembrolizumab (NCT03259867).

13.8 Perspectives

Recent preclinical and clinical findings have shed light on the impact of TACE on crucial entities such as tumor microenvironment, angiogenesis, and tumor-specific and innate immune responses. A better understanding of molecular pathways implicated in tumor physiology has led to design new combinatorial approaches to improve patients' outcomes. However, such a complex interconnected network of interacting molecules is difficult to depict and understand in the setting of patient's and cancer's heterogeneities. Thus, it is important to investigate the effect of TACE per se, not only locoregionally at the tissue level but also at the systemic level to gain knowledge on therapy and cancer-related molecular events to better select candidate drugs for combinatorial approaches with TACE.

Systemic antiangiogenic drugs have revolutionized the treatment of the advanced-stage HCC but are now being challenged by the new roller coaster in oncology: immunotherapy. The combination of systemic antiangiogenic drugs and immunotherapy is already successful, with bevacizumab combined with atezolizumab already being the new standard of care in first line [38]. Durvalumab/tremelimumab combination should be soon a second option for first-line therapy with announced superiority to sorafenib [51]. As of today, these combination studies mainly target the advanced- and intermediate-stage HCC patients, which are notoriously heterogeneous population, but the future might very well be to add local therapy to patients receiving systemic therapies.

Many ongoing trials combine TACE with a systemic immune checkpoint inhibitor. The next logical step would be to perform TACE with dual checkpoint inhibition as this regimen demonstrated to be superior to checkpoint inhibition monotherapy in some cancer type such as HCC or melanoma [67]. An anticipated limiting factor of dual checkpoint inhibition, in particular in the setting of liver cirrhosis, is toxicity. Another very appealing approach is to combine TACE with systemic immunotherapy and antiangiogenic therapy with many trials underway and results are very much expected.

Many components need to be investigated with this new approach of TACE combined with immunotherapy. In particular, fine-tuning will be needed with respect to the dose, timing (e.g., before vs. after TACE, concomitantly, sequentially), and duration of immunotherapy administration. The way TACE is done may impact outcomes and tumor antigen release, as it is not known if tumors subtotally treated may elicit a better immune response when compared to completely embolized ones. Additionally, the number and scheduling (on demand vs. scheduled) of TACEs in the setting of combined immunotherapy is to be defined.

Local drug delivery is a powerful approach in a treatment-resistant tumor such as HCC. TACE with drug-eluting beads loaded with antiangiogenic drugs combined with systemic immunotherapies is particularly appealing, and this approach should also be tested while the local administration of immunotherapies may prove to be beneficial.

In conclusion, the future of TACE in combination with systemic therapies is promising. Many approaches are currently being tested and hopefully will lead to better outcomes for patients and change the landscape of HCC therapy.

References

1. European Association for the Study of the Liver. Electronic address easl office easl office eu, European Association for the Study of the L. EASL Clinical Practice Guidelines: management of hepatocellular carcinoma. J Hepatol. 2018;69(1):182–236.

2. Frilling A, Clift AK. Therapeutic strategies for neuroendocrine liver metastases. Cancer. 2015;121(8):1172–86.
3. Lencioni R, Aliberti C, de Baere T, Garcia-Monaco R, Narayanan G, O'Grady E, et al. Transarterial treatment of colorectal cancer liver metastases with irinotecan-loaded drug-eluting beads: technical recommendations. J Vasc Interv Radiol. 2014;25(3):365–9.
4. Albert M, Kiefer MV, Sun W, Haller D, Fraker DL, Tuite CM, et al. Chemoembolization of colorectal liver metastases with cisplatin, doxorubicin, mitomycin C, ethiodol, and polyvinyl alcohol. Cancer. 2011;117(2):343–52.
5. Sahara S, Kawai N, Sato M, Tanaka T, Ikoma A, Nakata K, et al. Prospective evaluation of transcatheter arterial chemoembolization (TACE) with multiple anti-cancer drugs (epirubicin, cisplatin, mitomycin c, 5-fluorouracil) compared with TACE with epirubicin for treatment of hepatocellular carcinoma. Cardiovasc Interv Radiol. 2012;35(6):1363–71.
6. Duran R, Chapiro J, Schernthaner RE, Geschwind JF. Systematic review of catheter-based intra-arterial therapies in hepatocellular carcinoma: state of the art and future directions. Br J Radiol. 2015;88(1052):20140564.
7. Varela M, Real MI, Burrel M, Forner A, Sala M, Brunet M, et al. Chemoembolization of hepatocellular carcinoma with drug eluting beads: efficacy and doxorubicin pharmacokinetics. J Hepatol. 2007;46(3):474–81.
8. Takayasu K, Arii S, Ikai I, Kudo M, Matsuyama Y, Kojiro M, et al. Overall survival after transarterial lipiodol infusion chemotherapy with or without embolization for unresectable hepatocellular carcinoma: propensity score analysis. AJR Am J Roentgenol. 2010;194(3):830–7.
9. Degrauwe N, Hocquelet A, Digklia A, Schaefer N, Denys A, Duran R. Theranostics in interventional oncology: versatile carriers for diagnosis and targeted image-guided minimally invasive procedures. Front Pharmacol. 2019;10:450.
10. Lencioni R, de Baere T, Soulen MC, Rilling WS, Geschwind JF. Lipiodol transarterial chemoembolization for hepatocellular carcinoma: a systematic review of efficacy and safety data. Hepatology. 2016;64(1):106–16.
11. Harris AL. Hypoxia—a key regulatory factor in tumour growth. Nat Rev Cancer. 2002;2(1):38–47.
12. Wang GL, Jiang BH, Rue EA, Semenza GL. Hypoxia-inducible factor 1 is a basic-helix-loop-helix-PAS heterodimer regulated by cellular O2 tension. Proc Natl Acad Sci U S A. 1995;92(12):5510–4.
13. Poon RT, Lau C, Yu WC, Fan ST, Wong J. High serum levels of vascular endothelial growth factor predict poor response to transarterial chemoembolization in hepatocellular carcinoma: a prospective study. Oncol Rep. 2004;11(5):1077–84.
14. Sergio A, Cristofori C, Cardin R, Pivetta G, Ragazzi R, Baldan A, et al. Transcatheter arterial chemoembolization (TACE) in hepatocellular carcinoma (HCC): the role of angiogenesis and invasiveness. Am J Gastroenterol. 2008;103(4):914–21.
15. Shim JH, Park JW, Kim JH, An M, Kong SY, Nam BH, et al. Association between increment of serum VEGF level and prognosis after transcatheter arterial chemoembolization in hepatocellular carcinoma patients. Cancer Sci. 2008;99(10):2037–44.
16. Wang B, Xu H, Gao ZQ, Ning HF, Sun YQ, Cao GW. Increased expression of vascular endothelial growth factor in hepatocellular carcinoma after transcatheter arterial chemoembolization. Acta Radiol. 2008;49(5):523–9.
17. Ronald J, Nixon AB, Marin D, Gupta RT, Janas G, Chen W, et al. Pilot evaluation of angiogenesis Signaling factor response after transcatheter arterial embolization for hepatocellular carcinoma. Radiology. 2017;285(1):311–8.
18. Bize P, Duran R, Fuchs K, Dormond O, Namur J, Decosterd LA, et al. Antitumoral effect of sunitinib-eluting beads in the rabbit VX2 tumor model. Radiology. 2016;280(2):425–35.
19. Duran R, Namur J, Pascale F, Czuczman P, Bascal Z, Kilpatrick H, et al. Vandetanib-eluting radiopaque beads: pharmacokinetics, safety, and efficacy in a rabbit model of liver cancer. Radiology. 2019;293(3):695–703.
20. Vasudev NS, Reynolds AR. Anti-angiogenic therapy for cancer: current progress, unresolved questions and future directions. Angiogenesis. 2014;17(3):471–94.
21. Brown JM, Wilson WR. Exploiting tumour hypoxia in cancer treatment. Nat Rev Cancer. 2004;4(6):437–47.
22. Scheffer SR, Nave H, Korangy F, Schlote K, Pabst R, Jaffee EM, et al. Apoptotic, but not necrotic, tumor cell vaccines induce a potent immune response in vivo. Int J Cancer. 2003;103(2):205–11.
23. Festjens N, Vanden Berghe T, Vandenabeele P. Necrosis, a well-orchestrated form of cell demise: signalling cascades, important mediators and concomitant immune response. Biochim Biophys Acta. 2006;1757(9–10):1371–87.
24. Gamrekelashvili J, Kruger C, von Wasielewski R, Hoffmann M, Huster KM, Busch DH, et al. Necrotic tumor cell death in vivo impairs tumor-specific immune responses. J Immunol. 2007;178(3):1573–80.
25. Casares N, Pequignot MO, Tesniere A, Ghiringhelli F, Roux S, Chaput N, et al. Caspase-dependent immunogenicity of doxorubicin-induced tumor cell death. J Exp Med. 2005;202(12):1691–701.
26. Kroemer G, Galluzzi L, Kepp O, Zitvogel L. Immunogenic cell death in cancer therapy. Annu Rev Immunol. 2013;31:51–72.
27. Kim MJ, Jang JW, Oh BS, Kwon JH, Chung KW, Jung HS, et al. Change in inflammatory cytokine profiles after transarterial chemotherapy in patients with hepatocellular carcinoma. Cytokine. 2013;64(2):516–22.
28. Kohles N, Nagel D, Jungst D, Stieber P, Holdenrieder S. Predictive value of immunogenic cell death biomarkers HMGB1, sRAGE, and DNase in liver cancer patients receiving transarterial chemoembolization therapy. Tumour Biol. 2012;33(6):2401–9.

29. Ayaru L, Pereira SP, Alisa A, Pathan AA, Williams R, Davidson B, et al. Unmasking of alpha-fetoprotein-specific CD4(+) T cell responses in hepatocellular carcinoma patients undergoing embolization. J Immunol Baltim Md 1950. 2007;178(3):1914–22.
30. Nobuoka D, Motomura Y, Shirakawa H, Yoshikawa T, Kuronuma T, Takahashi M, et al. Radiofrequency ablation for hepatocellular carcinoma induces glypican-3 peptide-specific cytotoxic T lymphocytes. Int J Oncol. 2012;40(1):63–70.
31. Flecken T, Schmidt N, Hild S, Gostick E, Drognitz O, Zeiser R, et al. Immunodominance and functional alterations of tumor-associated antigen-specific CD8+ T-cell responses in hepatocellular carcinoma. Hepatology. 2014;59(4):1415–26.
32. Mizukoshi E, Nakamoto Y, Arai K, Yamashita T, Sakai A, Sakai Y, et al. Comparative analysis of various tumor-associated antigen-specific t-cell responses in patients with hepatocellular carcinoma. Hepatology. 2011;53(4):1206–16.
33. Li F, Guo Z, Lizee G, Yu H, Wang H, Si T. Clinical prognostic value of CD4+CD25+FOXP3+regulatory T cells in peripheral blood of Barcelona Clinic Liver Cancer (BCLC) stage B hepatocellular carcinoma patients. Clin Chem Lab Med. 2014;52(9):1357–65.
34. Liao J, Xiao J, Zhou Y, Liu Z, Wang C. Effect of transcatheter arterial chemoembolization on cellular immune function and regulatory T cells in patients with hepatocellular carcinoma. Mol Med Rep. 2015;12(4):6065–71.
35. Liao Y, Wang B, Huang ZL, Shi M, Yu XJ, Zheng L, et al. Increased circulating Th17 cells after transarterial chemoembolization correlate with improved survival in stage III hepatocellular carcinoma: a prospective study. PLoS One. 2013;8(4):e60444.
36. Cheng AL, Kang YK, Chen Z, Tsao CJ, Qin S, Kim JS, et al. Efficacy and safety of sorafenib in patients in the Asia-Pacific region with advanced hepatocellular carcinoma: a phase III randomised, double-blind, placebo-controlled trial. Lancet Oncol. 2009;10(1):25–34.
37. Llovet JM, Ricci S, Mazzaferro V, Hilgard P, Gane E, Blanc JF, et al. Sorafenib in advanced hepatocellular carcinoma. N Engl J Med. 2008;359(4):378–90.
38. Finn RS, Qin S, Ikeda M, Galle PR, Ducreux M, Kim TY, et al. Atezolizumab plus bevacizumab in unresectable hepatocellular carcinoma. N Engl J Med. 2020;382(20):1894–905.
39. Lencioni R, Kudo M, Ye SL, Bronowicki JP, Chen XP, Dagher L, et al. GIDEON (Global Investigation of therapeutic DEcisions in hepatocellular carcinoma and of its treatment with sorafeNib): second interim analysis. Int J Clin Pract. 2014;68(5):609–17.
40. Geschwind JF, Kudo M, Marrero JA, Venook AP, Chen XP, Bronowicki JP, et al. TACE treatment in patients with sorafenib-treated unresectable hepatocellular carcinoma in clinical practice: final analysis of GIDEON. Radiology. 2016;279(2):630–40.
41. Cai R, Song R, Pang P, Yan Y, Liao Y, Zhou C, et al. Transcatheter arterial chemoembolization plus sorafenib versus transcatheter arterial chemoembolization alone to treat advanced hepatocellular carcinoma: a meta-analysis. BMC Cancer. 2017;17(1):714.
42. Wang G, Liu Y, Zhou SF, Qiu P, Xu L, Wen P, et al. Sorafenib combined with transarterial chemoembolization in patients with hepatocellular carcinoma: a meta-analysis and systematic review. Hepatol Int. 2016;10(3):501–10.
43. Li L, Zhao W, Wang M, Hu J, Wang E, Zhao Y, et al. Transarterial chemoembolization plus sorafenib for the management of unresectable hepatocellular carcinoma: a systematic review and meta-analysis. BMC Gastroenterol. 2018;18(1):138.
44. Lencioni R, Llovet JM, Han G, Tak WY, Yang J, Guglielmi A, et al. Sorafenib or placebo plus TACE with doxorubicin-eluting beads for intermediate stage HCC: the SPACE trial. J Hepatol. 2016;64(5):1090–8.
45. Kudo M, Imanaka K, Chida N, Nakachi K, Tak WY, Takayama T, et al. Phase III study of sorafenib after transarterial chemoembolisation in Japanese and Korean patients with unresectable hepatocellular carcinoma. Eur J Cancer. 2011;47(14):2117–27.
46. Kudo M, Han G, Finn RS, Poon RT, Blanc JF, Yan L, et al. Brivanib as adjuvant therapy to transarterial chemoembolization in patients with hepatocellular carcinoma: a randomized phase III trial. Hepatology. 2014;60(5):1697–707.
47. Kudo M, Cheng AL, Park JW, Park JH, Liang PC, Hidaka H, et al. Orantinib versus placebo combined with transcatheter arterial chemoembolisation in patients with unresectable hepatocellular carcinoma (ORIENTAL): a randomised, double-blind, placebo-controlled, multicentre, phase 3 study. Lancet Gastroenterol Hepatol. 2018;3(1):37–46.
48. Pinter M, Ulbrich G, Sieghart W, Kolblinger C, Reiberger T, Li S, et al. Hepatocellular carcinoma: a phase II randomized controlled double-blind trial of transarterial chemoembolization in combination with biweekly intravenous administration of bevacizumab or a placebo. Radiology. 2015;277(3):903–12.
49. Park JW, Kim YJ, Kim DY, Bae SH, Paik SW, Lee YJ, et al. Sorafenib with or without concurrent transarterial chemoembolization in patients with advanced hepatocellular carcinoma: the phase III STAH trial. J Hepatol. 2019;70(4):684–91.
50. Ribas A, Wolchok JD. Cancer immunotherapy using checkpoint blockade. Science. 2018;359(6382):1350–5.
51. Kelley RK, Sangro B, Harris W, Ikeda M, Okusaka T, Kang YK, et al. Safety, efficacy, and pharmacodynamics of tremelimumab plus durvalumab for patients with unresectable hepatocellular carcinoma: randomized expansion of a phase I/II study. J Clin Oncol. 2021;39(27):2991–3001.
52. Shi L, Wang J, Ding N, Zhang Y, Zhu Y, Dong S, et al. Inflammation induced by incomplete radiofrequency ablation accelerates tumor progression and hinders PD-1 immunotherapy. Nat Commun. 2019;10(1):5421.

53. Duffy AG, Ulahannan SV, Makorova-Rusher O, Rahma O, Wedemeyer H, Pratt D, et al. Tremelimumab in combination with ablation in patients with advanced hepatocellular carcinoma. J Hepatol. 2017;66(3):545–51.
54. Pinato DJ, Cole T, Bengsch B, Tait P, Sayed AA, Abomeli F, et al. 750P—a phase Ib study of pembrolizumab following trans-arterial chemoembolization (TACE) in hepatocellular carcinoma (HCC): PETAL. Ann Oncol. 2019;30:v288.
55. Marabelle A, Tselikas L, de Baere T, Houot R. Intratumoral immunotherapy: using the tumor as the remedy. Ann Oncol. 2017;28:xii33-43.
56. Marabelle A, Andtbacka R, Harrington K, Melero I, Leidner R, de Baere T, et al. Starting the fight in the tumor: expert recommendations for the development of human intratumoral immunotherapy (HIT-IT). Ann Oncol. 2018;29(11):2163–74.
57. Tselikas L, Champiat S, Sheth RA, Yevich S, Ammari S, Deschamps F, et al. Interventional radiology for local immunotherapy in oncology. Clin Cancer Res. 2021;27(10):2698–705.
58. Yu J, Green MD, Li S, Sun Y, Journey SN, Choi JE, et al. Liver metastasis restrains immunotherapy efficacy via macrophage-mediated T cell elimination. Nat Med. 2021;27(1):152–64.
59. Sato T, Eschelman DJ, Gonsalves CF, Terai M, Chervoneva I, McCue PA, et al. Immunoembolization of malignant liver tumors, including uveal melanoma, using granulocyte-macrophage colony-stimulating factor. J Clin Oncol. 2008;26(33):5436–42.
60. Yamamoto A, Chervoneva I, Sullivan KL, Eschelman DJ, Gonsalves CF, Mastrangelo MJ, et al. High-dose immunoembolization: survival benefit in patients with hepatic metastases from Uveal Melanoma1. Radiology. 2009;252(1):290–8.
61. Valsecchi ME, Terai M, Eschelman DJ, Gonsalves CF, Chervoneva I, Shields JA, et al. Double-blinded, randomized phase II study using embolization with or without granulocyte-macrophage colony-stimulating factor in uveal melanoma with hepatic metastases. J Vasc Interv Radiol. 2015;26(4):523–32 e2.
62. Wilson WR, Hay MP. Targeting hypoxia in cancer therapy. Nat Rev Cancer. 2011;11(6):393–410.
63. Li Y, Zhao L, Li XF. The hypoxia-activated prodrug TH-302: exploiting hypoxia in cancer therapy. Front Pharmacol. 2021;12:636892.
64. Duran R, Mirpour S, Pekurovsky V, Ganapathy-Kanniappan S, Brayton CF, Cornish TC, et al. Preclinical benefit of hypoxia-activated intra-arterial therapy with evofosfamide in liver cancer. Clin Cancer Res. 2017;23(2):536–48.
65. Lin WH, Yeh SH, Yeh KH, Chen KW, Cheng YW, Su TH, et al. Hypoxia-activated cytotoxic agent tirapazamine enhances hepatic artery ligation-induced killing of liver tumor in HBx transgenic mice. Proc Natl Acad Sci USA. 2016;113(42):11937–42.
66. Abi-Jaoudeh N, Dayyani F, Chen PJ, Fernando D, Fidelman N, Javan H, et al. Phase I trial on arterial embolization with hypoxia activated tirapazamine for unresectable hepatocellular carcinoma. J Hepatocell Carcinoma. 2021;8:421–34.
67. Postow MA, Chesney J, Pavlick AC, Robert C, Grossmann K, McDermott D, et al. Nivolumab and ipilimumab versus ipilimumab in untreated melanoma. N Engl J Med. 2015;372(21):2006–17.

TACE Side Effects and Complications

14

Pier Giorgio Nardis, Leonardo Teodoli, Bianca Rocco, Simone Ciaglia, and Carlo Catalano

14.1 Side Effects: Post-Embolization Syndrome (PES)

Patients undergoing TACE can experience post-embolization syndrome in up to 80%. PES symptoms include fever, pain, nausea, and vomiting, typically occurring within the first 48–72 hours after embolization.

Etiology PES is assumed to be mediated by inflammatory cytokines released as a result of embolization-induced cells's necrosis and/or chemotherapeutic agents. Incidence of PES in patients who underwent transarterial embolization (TAE) is similar to the one reported in patients treated with TACE, implying that the mechanism of PES is probably driven by liver necrosis due to interruption of blood flow, rather than by chemotherapeutic agents.

The severity of PES depends on the branch level of chemoembolization: The more extensive embolization is performed, the greater the possibility of PES manifestation. In theory, superselective embolization in selected cases will allow avoidance of PES and could reduce the discomfort of seriously ill patients.

Symptoms TACE-related PES is often mild and self-limited. It can appear immediately, afterward, or during 10 days following the procedure, prolonging hospitalization and limiting the application of additional treatments. Symptoms can be fever, abdominal pain, nausea and/or vomiting, and elevated transaminase levels.

Identification of preoperative predictors of PES is challenging. Some significant predictors of protracted recovery risk factors reported in literature are previous PES and large tumor burden. Interestingly, age, individual laboratory values, multiple TACE procedures, model for end-stage liver disease score, Child-Turcotte-Pugh class, and albumin-bilirubin ratio grade are insensitive to PES.

Identification of PES predictors is important to suggest alternative therapies or prophylactic medications to prevent symptoms in high-risk populations. Some studies identified female sex and alcohol-related HCC as potential risk factors for developing PES in patients undergoing TACE.

Treatment There is no standard treatment or premedication to prevent post-embolization syndrome.

Symptomatic medication includes use of anti-emetic drugs (mostly 5HT3 antagonist) and analgesics.

P. G. Nardis (✉) · L. Teodoli · B. Rocco · S. Ciaglia · C. Catalano
Vascular and Interventional Radiology Unit, Department of Radiological, Oncological, and Anatomo-Pathological Sciences, Sapienza University of Rome, Rome, Italy
e-mail: carlo.catalano@uniroma1.it

P. Lucatelli (ed.), *Transarterial Chemoembolization (TACE)*,
https://doi.org/10.1007/978-3-031-36261-3_14

Recent studies suggests that dexamethasone, in adjunction to the mixture of Lipiodol and chemotherapeutic agent or as premedication in DEM-TACE, reduces significantly PES [1–10].

14.2 Complications

While side effects of TACE are common, complications of TACE are rare and their frequency is lower than 5%.

The incidence of complications increases with the severity of the underlying clinical status of the patient and the duration of the procedure.

Some risk factors such as portal vein obstruction, impaired liver functional reserve, biliary obstruction, previous biliary surgery, excessive administration of embolic agent, and nonselective embolization increase complication rate.

Thirty-day mortality rate following complications ranges from 1% to 4%.

Diagnosis of complications is based on signs and symptoms, laboratory testing, imaging evaluation, or interventional procedures. The imaging assessment includes contrast-enhanced computed tomography (CT) scan, magnetic resonance imaging (MRI), or ultrasound [10].

14.2.1 Early Complications

14.2.1.1 Intraprocedural Complications

Vascular Complications

Access Site Complications: Puncture Site Hematoma and Pseudoaneurysm

Vascular access site complications range from 0.44% to 4% according to the type of the procedure, therefore depending on the size of the sheath. Common femoral artery at the femoral head is the most appropriate vascular access because of the diameter and the location allowing appropriate compression and hemostasis. It is well known that puncture below the femoral head can produce hematoma or pseudoaneurysm at the root ofh the thigh due to inadequate compression site while puncture above the femoral head and inguinal ligament can cause retroperitoneal bleeding. The use of ultrasound guidance allows accurate location of the puncture site, avoiding plaque and arterial branches; moreover, the monoparietal puncture approach significantly reduces the complication rate [10–13].

Using smaller size catheters (5 French or smaller) may reduce the risk of complications.

Reversal of anticoagulation to baseline status by monitoring activated clotting time can minimize this risk.

The most common complication of femoral artery puncture is groin hematoma that is generally self-limiting and does not require further treatment.

In cases of uncontrolled hematoma or pseudoaneurysm, treatment is recommended including groin compression, thrombin injection, surgical evacuation of the hematoma, and arterial suturing [14, 15].

In recent years, radial access is becoming the standard approach to perform TACE in many centers, thus reducing further incidence of vascular site complications and improving patient comfort during post-procedural period [16, 17].

Catheterism-Related Complication

- **Spasm** of the hepatic artery after TACE is rare and the reason for which is unknown. The use of small size catheters and selective catheterization with microcatheters reduces significantly the incidence of vascular spasm. The spasm of the hepatic artery is related to the mechanical stimulation of the hepatic artery by the guide and catheters. In addition, the hepatic artery damage caused by chemotherapeutic drugs and embolic agents may also be relevant to the arterial spasm [18]. Generally, selective infusion of nitroglycerin and lidocaine can successfully treat vascular spasm.
- **Hepatic artery dissection:** Vascular dissection is an uncommon complication, and it is generally due to vessel wall trauma by catheter and guide manipulation (Fig. 14.1). In the elderly patients, atherosclerosis is an additional risk factor for vascular dissection. In the majority of cases of hepatic artery or its

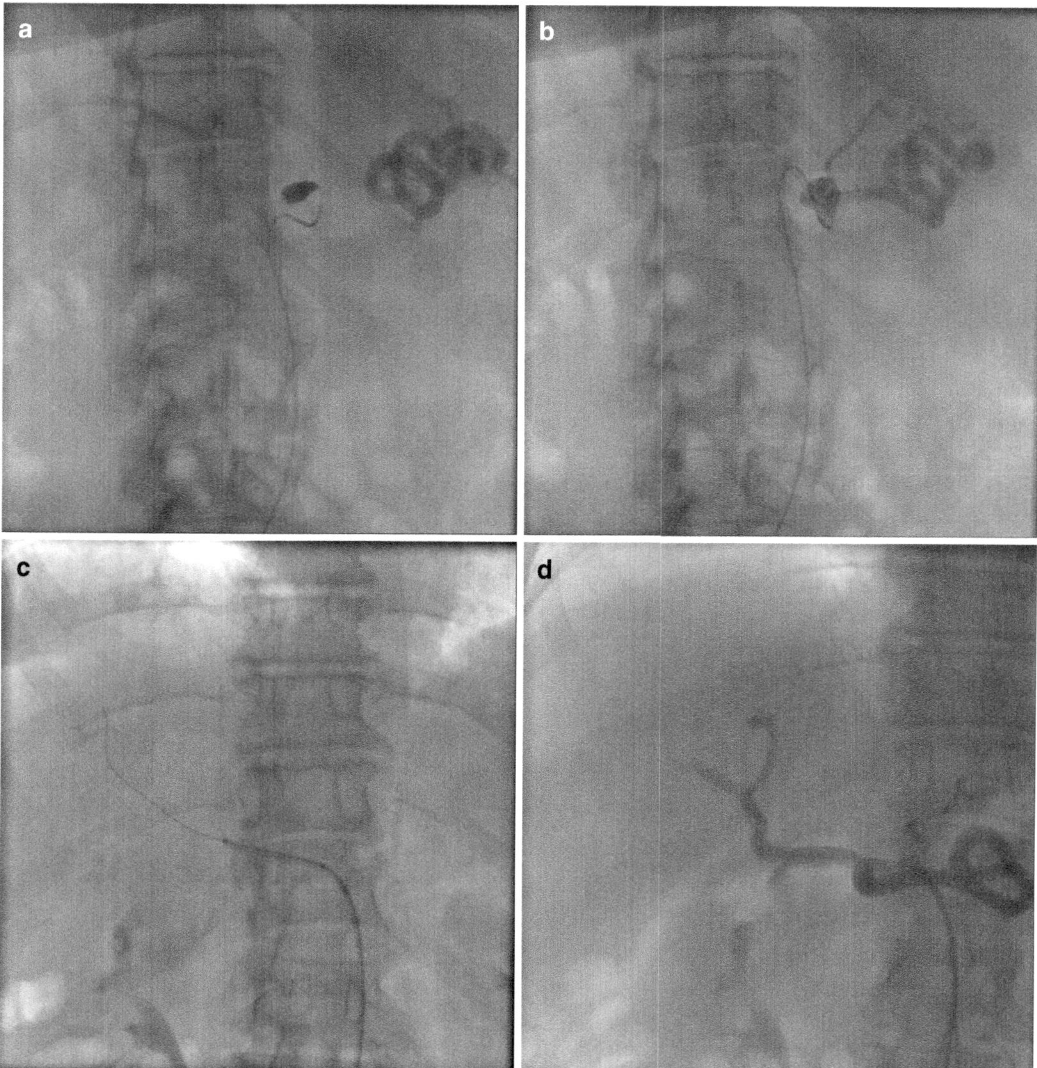

Fig. 14.1 (**a**, **b**) Hepatic artery dissection and occlusion during selective catheterization. (**c**, **d**) Hepatic artery dissection crossing and ballooning with flow restoration

branches dissections, no additional treatment is required since no flow limitation is observed. In some cases of flow-limiting dissection, gently ballooning or stenting of the dissection is necessary [19, 20].

- **Intra-arterial thrombosis** can be secondary to spasm or dissections and treatment depends on the etiology. Heparinization reduces risk of thrombosis [13, 15].
- **Arteritis** is a rare complication of TACE that can affect the main hepatic artery or its secondary branches with final evolution characterized by occlusion due to thrombosis. Severe stenosis of the hepatic artery is usually easily compensated by collaterals, but this complication can make successive TACE impossible. Wall injury develops early during treatment, and probably depends on a direct acute toxic effect of the chemotherapy agent itself, rather than mechanical wall injury due to repeated catheterizations. Risk factors include proximal administration of embolic agent, multiple

procedures, time interval of less than 1–2 months between procedures, use of Lipiodol, and nonuse of microcatheter [2, 21].

14.2.1.2 Post-Procedural Complications

Nontarget Embolization

Gastrointestinal Embolization

Post-TACE gastric lesions are due to the backflow of embolic materials into the gastric artery with a subsequent reduction in gastric mucosal blood flow, which may cause gastric complications such as ulceration or perforation. Anatomical variations, such as right gastric artery branching distally from proper hepatic artery or from its branches or the accessory left gastric artery arising from the left hepatic artery, are most likely associated with higher incidence of post-TACE gastric lesions and should be carefully researched during angiography [22].

Acute Lung Injury

This complication is rare (0.05%). Acute lung injury or respiratory distress syndrome is caused by the embolic material that reaches the pulmonary vascularization, mostly because of intratumoral arteriovenous shunt with consequent chemical injury caused by infused chemotherapeutic drug and embolizing agent. Patients present dyspnea, cough, expectoration, decrease in blood oxygen saturation within 24–48 hours after TACE, elevated D-dimer, diffuse pulmonary infiltration, and accumulation of Lipiodol (in case of conventional TACE) on post-procedural chest CT scan.

Several risk factors including preexisting chronic respiratory disease, hepatic arteriovenous fistula, large hypervascular HCC (>10 cm) with arteriovenous shunts, large-volume Lipiodol administration (>14.5 mL), and trans-inferior phrenic artery embolization have been identified to develop acute lung injury after TACE. While extremely rare, other chemoembolization agent may also have potential for induction of acute lung injury. The ideal management strategy for TACE-associated acute lung injury includes oxygenation, systemic corticosteroids administration, and lung protective ventilation according to the severity of symptoms [1, 23, 24].

Spinal Cord Injury

Spinal cord injury is an extremely rare but severe complication of TACE. This fearsome complication often occurs in patients with parasitic vascularization of HCC, especially by intercostal arteries [25].

An intercostal artery collateral blood supply usually occurs in advanced HCC or after multiple sessions of TACE. The intercostal arteries frequently involved in supplying HCCs are T10, T9, and T11, in order of decreasing association. Paraplegia may result from the unintended embolization of spinal branches arising from intercostal or lumbar collateral vessels.

The risk of spinal cord injury associated with intercostal artery intervention exists because spinal cord arteries derive from the proximal tract of intercostal arteries. The spinal cord is supplied primarily by one anterior and two posterior spinal arteries, which are augmented by radicular arteries derived from spinal branches of cervical, intercostal, and lumbar arteries. The anterior spinal artery supplies blood to the anterior two-thirds of the cord, including the anterior horns of the gray matter, spinothalamic tracts, and corticospinal tracts, which primarily control the motor nuclei. The two posterior spinal arteries supply the dorsal columns and the posterior horns, which mostly process sensory information. Therefore, because of anatomy and neurological distribution, the embolic materials may bring about an embolic event with possible serious manifestations, even though the blood supply network of the spinal cord includes multiple anastomoses [26–28].

Acute Cholecystitis

Acute cholecystitis has been reported to occur after TACE with an incidence of 1.5–4.9%. Cholecystitis and gallbladder infarction are often detected in patients treated with TACE. The two events are essentially the manifestations of one disease at two different stages. If the earlier cholecystitis cannot be reversed, it will consequently progress into gallbladder necrosis. The clinical manifestations generally include fever and abdominal pain, the same as for common cholecystitis. While acute cholecystitis can usually be resolved with conservative therapy in case of infarcted gallbladder, a cholecystectomy is mandatory. The prognosis will be very good with rapid treatment. The blood supply to the gallbladder derives from the cystic artery and if present from accessory cystic artery, both can arise from the right, or the left, or even from the common hepatic artery. Therefore, the gallbladder can be embolized by the refluxed embolic materials for anatomical and/or technical causes, even though the location of the hepatic arterial catheter is as distal to the cystic artery as possible.

Some interventional radiologists prophylactically embolize with metal coils the cystic artery proximally in order to avoid embolizing agent migration into the cystic artery; however, the evidence of this practice is uncertain [18].

Cutaneous Embolization

Vaso-occlusive manifestations of the skin is a rare complication of TACE. In some patients, the feeder of the hepatic nodule has small collateral arteries that cannot be avoided or recognized during angiography. One of these collateral arteries is the hepatic falciform artery, which is incidentally seen on angiography in 2–24.5% of cases. The hepatic falciform artery runs in the falciform ligament and in turn supplies subcutaneous tissue around the umbilicus. Occlusion of the hepatic falciform artery by the embolic agent can result in skin infarction and necrosis.

Treatment consists of oral nonsteroidal anti-inflammatory agents, and usually, the skin lesions resolve within a year from the procedure. Prophylactic application of ice could potentially prevent cutaneous complications of nontarget chemoembolization. It is recommended to place the tip of the microcatheter distal to the origin of the hepatic falciform artery. While prophylactic falciform artery embolization has been advised, its efficacy is controversial [29].

Pancreatic Embolization

Acute pancreatitis, as result of nontarget embolization, is an uncommon (0.9–2%) but serious complication.

The diagnosis of acute pancreatitis is proven mainly according to raises of serum amylase and lipase levels, abdominal pain, and other symptoms such as fever, fatigue, and vomiting. Most of these abnormal findings occurred within 24 h after TACE. Re-elevation of pancreatic enzymes predicts worsening of the pancreatitis. In some cases, a pancreatic injury can develop into a necrotizing pancreatitis that may be lethal when sepsis and multiorgan failure occurs.

Symptomatic acute pancreatitis is caused by embolic material into the pancreatic-duodenal artery, occluding a large peripheral portion of the pancreatic vascular bed, leading to ischemia of the pancreas.

Some authors reported an association between the frequency of this complication and the type and volume of the particles used for the embolization: Serum amylase activity increased slightly in patients treated with Lipiodol and Gelfoam powder.

To prevent this complication, care has to be taken during the injection of embolic material in order to avoid reflux in the gastroduodenal artery [1, 22, 30, 31].

14.2.2 Late Complications

14.2.2.1 Biliary Complication

The incidence of biliary strictures is generally low after TACE, ranging from 0.5% to 10%. The incidence of biliary complications is due to the exclusive vascularization of the bile duct by the hepatic artery. This can cause necrosis of the bile duct, ectasia, the formation of bilomas, or stenosis [32]. Predisposing factors include tumor size, dilation of the bile duct prior to the procedure, proximal embolization, less than 3 months interval between two procedures, and the injection of Lipiodol or the use of small particles. DEM-TACE is associated with an increased bile duct damage compared with c-TACE, but this finding is rather controversial [33].

Patients with advanced cirrhosis have a lower risk of developing locoregional toxicity due to gradual hypertrophy of the peribiliary vascular plexus caused by portal hypertension and collateral vascularization.

When the biliary wall damage caused by embolization causes necrosis, biloma can appear, although usually asymptomatic. The reported incidence of intrahepatic biloma is very low and can be observed as hypodense areas on CT close to the treated lesion.

Development of biliary strictures can have minimal clinical manifestations in case of peripheral branch involvement; however, consequences can be severe in case of central or diffuse strictures, resulting in hyperbilirubinemia that can be associated with cholangitis. Although the clinical symptoms rarely present, the laboratory-tested values of serum alkaline phosphatase, gamma-glutamyl transpeptidase, and leucine aminopeptidase increase gradually over approximately 1 month following the procedure. US examination for dilation of the bile duct in the liver is able to confirm the diagnosis. Patients with this complication can be systemically treated with antibiotics. The treatments vary according to the severity of the complication, ranging from conservative treatment, antibiotics regimen to biliary drainage [1, 18, 32–36].

14.2.2.2 Liver Abscess

Liver abscess formation after TACE for hepatic tumors is a rare but serious complication with substantial morbidity and mortality. The incidence of abscess formation after TACE varies from 0.2% to 2%. In most patients, abscesses present as solitary lesions (66.7%), and the imaging test of choice is CT (Fig. 14.2).

After TACE, tumors become partly or completely necrotic, which serves as an ideal pabulum for bacterial growth. The locally immunosuppressive effects of any chemotherapeutic agent used during TACE and the lack of perfusion after embolization that reduces the efficacy of systemic antibiotics play a central role in the susceptibility for abscess formation. Also, as discussed above, embolotherapy can result in disruption of the bile duct wall, permitting direct intercommunication of the luminal contents with the necrotic tissue.

The risk factors associated with this complication are biliointestinal bypass, advanced age, diabetes mellitus, tumor size, and portal vein occlusion.

Several studies reported that liver abscess may be unavoidable if the sphincter of Oddi has been compromised either by a hepatojejunostomy or biliary tube or stent. Typically, bile is sterile; however, in patients with bilioenteric anastomosis or with prior sphincterotomy or biliary stenting, the biliary tree is colonized by enteric

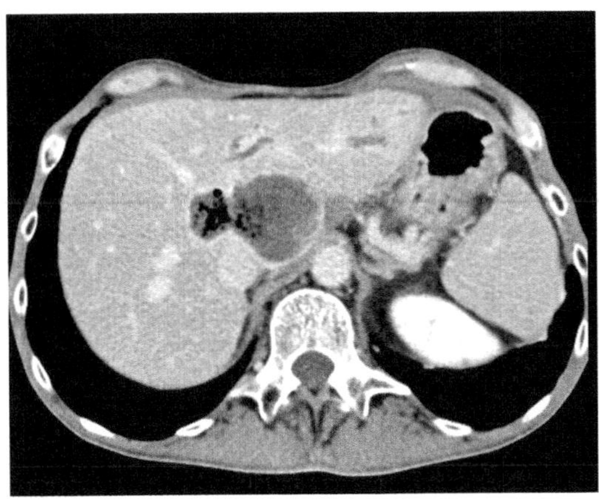

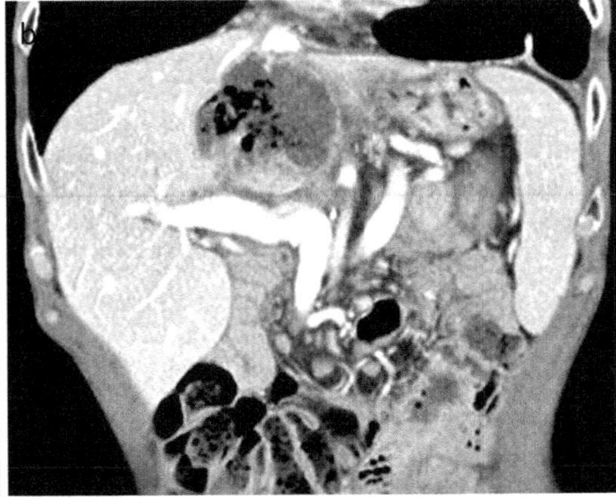

Fig. 14.2 (**a**, **b**) Large liver abscess following selective TACE in patient with bilioenteric anastomosis

bacteria; most authors have shown that an incompetent or absent sphincter of Oddi has been shown to convey a very high risk of subsequent abscess development after TACE, with an incidence of up to 86%.

Other possible risk factors correlated with the development of liver abscess include patient and tumor characteristics such as leukopenia, immunodeficiency, and diabetes mellitus. With regard to technical aspects of c-TACE, embolization using absorbable gelatin sponge or visualization of oily portogram during embolization correlates with a significantly elevated risk of development of liver abscess.

The effectiveness of prophylaxis in this setting is unproven, although several clinical series have advised that major infectious complications may be sustained in this population. Many operators routinely administer antibiotic prophylaxis before TACE, including coverage for skin flora and for gram-negative enteric organisms, even though this practice has not been prospectively verified to be of benefit for all patients. The risk of post-embolization infection appears to be reduced by the performance of a bowel preparation the night before treatment and by ensuring coverage of gram-positive and gram-negative aerobic and anaerobic organisms [37].

The incidence of liver abscesses is extremely reduced by administering a high dose of antibiotic dissolved in the embolizing particles allowing high concentration of antibiotic in the necrotic area, thus reducing the probability of developing a bacterial infection. Abscesses measuring less than 5 cm may be treatable with antibiotics, and percutaneous or surgical drainage is the preferred option in cases greater than 5 cm. Liver abscesses are notoriously difficult to treat and may require prolonged drainage, repeat drainage, and long-term antibiotics [1, 6, 36, 38–41].

14.2.2.3 Hepatic Infarction

The development of hepatic infarction is a severe complication detected with a low incidence. Clinical symptoms are mainly abdominal pain and fever, with clear and quick rises of the levels of serum total bilirubin, alanine aminotransaminase, aspartate aminotransferase, and C-reactive protein. Diagnosis can be made based on the subsequent CT scan. Extensive liver necrosis can be lethal while segmental or lobar infarction can result in very serious complications such as liver abscess and sepsis. Most cases of hepatic necrosis are complicated by infection, in particular those caused by gram-negative bacteria. Therefore, prophylactic antibiotics should be administered to prevent septic complications if a liver infarct is supposed. Treatment options for infected hepatic necrosis include administration of intravenous antibiotics, percutaneous drainage, and open surgical drainage or liver resection or even minimally invasive techniques such as laparoscopic necrosectomy for the hepatic debridement. Once the common percutaneous drainage fails to relieve the infected hepatic necrosis, surgical necrosectomy will be necessary.

Major portal vein obstruction is a well-known risk factor for liver infarction after TACE. Consequently, in patients with major portal vein obstruction, TACE should be carefully considered with reduced amounts of chemoembolic agents selectively directed into the tumor-feeding arteries. In addition, the preoperative liver function of the patient has a great influence on the incidence and outcome of hepatic infarction [5, 18, 42].

14.2.2.4 Tumor and Hepatic Rupture

The reported incidence of hepatic rupture is 0.6%. The risk factors for hepatic rupture are large tumor (>10 cm) or tumors located on the liver surface.

Tumor rupture following TACE is a rare but potentially lethal complication due to massive hemorrhage. The interval between the treatment and rupture varies between different cases. The complication happened mainly after the first treatment.

The mechanism of rupture of HCC after TACE is uncertain. It can be assumed to be connected to tumor necrosis and increased pressure due to oedema inside the tumor after TACE. Male patients are at higher risk of rupture for indeterminate reasons.

Rupture of the HCC should be suspected when the patient complains of abdominal pain associated with hemodynamic changes, a drop in hemoglobin concentration of 2 g/dL or more, and diagnosis of hemoperitoneum verified by abdominal paracentesis or CT scan. Management of patients with rupture of HCC following TACE is difficult as most of them have already been diagnosed as having large, inoperable tumors and impaired liver function. Although there have been many reports of treatments for extrahepatic rupture of HCC, only a few are about tumor rupture after TACE, which indicated that its outcome is often self-limited and that the patients can survive to the hemodynamic and liver function insult without any interventional procedure. Conservative management can be performed while in some cases, mass embolization is indicated [18].

14.2.2.5 Renal Function Decline

The reported incidence of this complication is 0.6%. With regard to renal function decline (defined as a sudden increase in creatinine greater than 50% over the baseline level or more than 1.5 mg/dL within the first 7 days after the procedure), the underlying mechanism is contrast-induced nephrotoxicity, although it is true that the rate of renal decline is higher in patients with HCC who undergo TACE than other angiographic procedure. The risk of renal failure is related to the dose and number of sessions of TACE and may have a cumulative effect on this risk [1].

In literature, only few papers show correlation about contrast-induced nephropathy (CIN) and TACE while several studies examined the incidence of CIN after percutaneous coronary intervention or contrast-enhanced CT. Some risk factors have been identified for CIN such as chronic kidney disease, diabetes mellitus, advanced age, hypovolemia, hypotension, heart failure, contrast media volume, and use of nephrotoxic drugs.

A recent study estimated the incidence of CIN as 4.6%. Tumor size bigger than 5 cm and lower serum albumin level were discovered as independent risk factors of CIN in patients who underwent TACE.

Use of low-osmolality contrast agents, reducing of the amount of contrast, and using nephron protectants prior to TACE may help reduce the risk of renal failure [1, 43, 44]. Adequate hydration is recommended, although there are different protocols in the literature and it should be considered not to overhydrate the cirrhotic patient, favoring fluids with low osmotic fluids [43, 45–47].

14.2.2.6 Hepatic Failure

Hepatic function decline can be found in almost all patients after TACE: Transient hepatic dysfunction happens in the majority of cases and the majority of patients recover spontaneously with or without supportive treatment.

However, the long-term and irreversible weakening of liver function that develops in the residual patients could barely be inverted by clinical treatments, which results in acute liver failure in about half of the patients.

Irreversible worsening of liver function or even acute liver failure can be often found in patients with severe loss of functional reserve (Child-Pugh advanced class B or C) that existed prior to the treatment. Another factor that may affect the TACE-related hepatic function damage is portal venous obstruction. Although it has been established that TACE did not cause serious damage to liver function with preserved hepatic functional reserve, hepatic insufficiency after TACE was much more likely to arise in patients with portal venous obstruction.

The reactivation of HBV can play a fundamental role in some cases of hepatic failure. The percentage of HBV reactivation in chronic HBV carriers receiving systemic chemotherapy is similar to those in patients who underwent TACE and reported to be 19–55%. The mechanism of HBV reactivation during chemotherapy has not been completely understood. Hypothetically, immunosuppressive or cytotoxic mediators increase HBV replication, leading to widespread hepatocyte infection with the viruses. When these drugs are withdrawn, restoration of immune function results in rapid destruction of infected hepatocytes. In addition, it was reported that various chemotherapeutic agents were associated with viral reactivation and precore/core mutations might play an important role [18, 38].

The reported incidence of ascitic decompensation after TACE is 2.8%. The development of early ascites is negatively associated with the overall survival of compensated patients treated with TACE.

This finding is related to low albumin, low hemoglobin, and prior episodes of clinical ascites. The presence of significant portal hypertension and/or worse liver function might imply that patients are inclined to complications in chemoembolization procedures and to the consequent impairment in overall survival. The development of ascites after TACE is independent of the radiological response (the overall survival rate is similar in patients who developed ascites, indicating that this is not associated with tumor development) [18].

The diagnosis of liver failure is based on clinical manifestations, including slight jaundice and associated debilitation and/or dyspepsia several days after TACE. Some serious cases may show severe jaundice and ascitic fluid and even hepatic encephalopathy, with the most serious case developing into acute hepatic dysfunction following death. The only intervention possible is symptomatic support: IV hydration, pressure support, and medical therapies for encephalopathy may help stabilize the patient until the liver recovers.

For some selected patients with acute liver failure, orthotopic liver transplantation might represent the best treatment option.

References

1. Marcacuzco Quinto A, et al. Complications of transarterial chemoembolization (TACE) in the treatment of liver Tumors. Cirugía Española (English Edition). 2018;96(9):560–7. https://doi.org/10.1016/j.cireng.2018.10.017.
2. Szemitko M, Golubinska-Szemitko E, Wilk-Milczarek E, Falkowski A. Side effect/complication risk related to injection branch level of chemoembolization in treatment of metastatic liver lesions from colorectal cancer. J Clin Med. 2020;10(1):121. https://doi.org/10.3390/jcm10010121.
3. Khalaf MH, et al. A predictive model for postembolization syndrome after transarterial hepatic chemoembolization of hepatocellular carcinoma. Radiology. 2019;290(1):254–61. https://doi.org/10.1148/radiol.2018180257.
4. Piscaglia F, Tovoli F, Pini P, Salvatore V. A new horizon in the prevention of the postembolization syndrome after transcatheter arterial chemoembolization for hepatocellular carcinoma. Hepatology. 67:2. John Wiley and Sons Inc., pp. 467–469, Feb. 01, 2018. https://doi.org/10.1002/hep.29517.
5. Clark TWI. Complications of hepatic chemoembolization. Semin Interv Radiol. 2006;23(2):119–25. https://doi.org/10.1055/s-2006-941442.
6. Ogasawara S, et al. A randomized placebo-controlled trial of prophylactic dexamethasone for transcatheter arterial chemoembolization. Hepatology. 2018;67(2):575–85. https://doi.org/10.1002/hep.29403.
7. Agrawal R, et al. Identifying predictors and evaluating the role of steroids in the prevention of post-embolization syndrome after transarterial chemoembolization and bland embolization. Ann Gastroenterol. 2021;34(2):241–6. https://doi.org/10.20524/aog.2020.0566.
8. Leung DA, Goin JE, Sickles C, Raskay BJ, and Soulen MC Determinants of postembolization syndrome after hepatic chemoembolization. J Vasc Interv Radiol. 2001;2(3):321–6. https://doi.org/10.1016/s1051-0443(07)61911-3.
9. Lo CM, et al. Randomized controlled trial of transarterial Lipiodol chemoembolization for unresectable hepatocellular carcinoma. Hepatology. 2002;35(5):1164–71. https://doi.org/10.1053/jhep.2002.33156.
10. Tu J, et al. The incidence and outcome of major complication following conventional TAE/TACE for hepatocellular carcinoma. Medicine (United States). 2016;95(49):e5606. https://doi.org/10.1097/MD.0000000000005606.
11. Grier D, Hartnell G. Percutaneous femoral artery puncture: practice and anatomy. 1990. Br J Radiol. 1990;63(752): 602–4. https://doi.org/10.1259/0007-1285-63-752-602.
12. Rapoport S, Snidemman KW, Morse SS, Proto MH, and Glenn Ross RR. TECHNICAL DEVELOPMENTS AND INSTRUMENTATION pseudoaneurysm: a complication of faulty technique in femoral arterial puncture.
13. Siiber S. Rapid hemostasis of arterial puncture sites with collagen in patients undergoing diagnostic and interventional cardiac catheterization. 1997.
14. Percutaneous injection of thrombin for the treatment of pseudoaneurysms after catheterization: an alternative to sonographically guided compression. [Online]. Available: www.ajronline.org
15. Formanek G, Frech RS, and Amplatz K. Arterial thrombus formation during clinical percutaneous catheterization. [Online]. Available: http://circ.ahajournals.org/

16. Toyoda H, et al. Safety, feasibility, and comfort of hepatic angiography and transarterial intervention with radial access for hepatocellular carcinoma. JGH Open. 2021;5(9):1041–6. https://doi.org/10.1002/jgh3.12628.
17. Du N, et al. Transradial access chemoembolization for hepatocellular carcinoma in comparation with transfemoral access. Transl Cancer Res. 2019;8:1795–805. https://doi.org/10.21037/tcr.2019.08.40.
18. Sun Z, et al. Hepatic and biliary damage after transarterial chemoembolization for malignant hepatic tumors: incidence, diagnosis, treatment, outcome and mechanism. Crit Rev Oncol Hematol. 2011;79(2):164–74. https://doi.org/10.1016/j.critrevonc.2010.07.019.
19. Goh WXT, et al. Management of arterial dissections in 12 patients during transarterial chemoembolization and yttrium-90 selective internal radiotherapy for primary and secondary liver tumours. Abdom Radiol. 2021;46(4):1737–45. https://doi.org/10.1007/s00261-020-02810-1.
20. Belli AM, Markose G, Morgan R. The role of interventional radiology in the management of abdominal visceral artery aneurysms. Cardiovasc Intervent Radiol. 2012;35(2):234–43. https://doi.org/10.1007/s00270-011-0201-3.
21. Iii HMR, Silberzweig JE, Mitty HA, Lou WYW, Ahn J, and Cooper JM. Hepatic arterial complications in liver transplant recipients treated with pretransplantation chemoembolization for hepatocellular carcinoma. Radiology. 2000;214(3):775–9. https://doi.org/10.1148/radiology.214.3.r00mr31775.
22. Yamaguchi T, et al. Acute necrotizing pancreatitis as a fatal complication following DC bead transcatheter arterial chemoembolization for hepatocellular carcinoma: a case report and review of the literature. Mol Clini Oncol. 2018; https://doi.org/10.3892/mco.2018.1690.
23. Fang L-J, Chen L-Y, Sun J-H, and Zhou J-Y. Clinical characteristics and outcomes of acute lung injury caused by transcatheter arterial chemoembolization for hepatocellular carcinoma: a retrospective cohort study from a single institution in China. 2019.
24. Ruan JY, Lin JT, Xiong Y, Chen ZZ, Chen JH, Yu HJ. Clinical characteristics of transarterial chemoembolization in treatment of primary hepatocellular carcinoma complicated with respiratory distress syndrome. Technol Cancer Res Treat. 2020;19 https://doi.org/10.1177/1533033820970673.
25. Lin GH, Shih YL. Paraplegia following transarterial chemoembolisation for hepatocellular carcinoma: a case report. Acta Chir Belg. 2020; https://doi.org/10.1080/00015458.2020.1726097.
26. Park SJ, et al. Spinal cord injury after conducting transcatheter arterial chemoembolization for costal metastasis of hepatocellular carcinoma. Clin Mol Hepatol. 2012;18(3):316–20. https://doi.org/10.3350/cmh.2012.18.3.316.
27. Bazine A, et al. Spinal cord ischemia secondary to transcatheter arterial chemoembolization for hepatocellular carcinoma. Case Rep Gastroenterol. 2014;8(3):264–9. https://doi.org/10.1159/000368075.
28. Kim HC, Jin WC, Lee W, Hwan JJ, Jae HP. Recognizing extrahepatic collateral vessels that supply hepatocellular carcinoma to avoid complications of transcatheter arterial chemoembolization. Radiographics. 2005;25(SPEC. ISS) https://doi.org/10.1148/rg.25si055508.
29. Kuan A, Khoo L. Retiform Purpura as a complication of microsphere emboli following transarterial chemoembolization for primary hepatocellular carcinoma: a case report and literature review CASE REPORT. 2019. [Online]. Available: www.amjdermatopathology.com |1.
30. Tan Y, Sheng J, Tan H, Mao J. Pancreas lipiodol embolism induced acute necrotizing pancreatitis following transcatheter arterial chemoembolization for hepatocellular carcinoma: a case report and literature review. Medicine (United States). 2019;98:48. Lippincott Williams and Wilkins, Nov. 01. https://doi.org/10.1097/MD.0000000000018095.
31. Alcívar-Vásquez JM, Ontanilla-Clavijo G, Ferrer-Ríos MT, and Pascasio-Acevedo JM. Letters to the Editor Acute necrotizing pancreatitis after transarterial chemoembolization of hepatocellular carcinoma: an usual complication. 2014. Rev Esp Enferm Dig. 2014;106(2):147–9. https://doi.org/10.4321/s1130-01082014000200014.
32. Dhamija E, Paul SB, Gamanagatti SR, Acharya SK. Biliary complications of arterial chemoembolization of hepatocellular carcinoma. Diagn Interv Imaging. 2015;96(11):1169–75. https://doi.org/10.1016/j.diii.2015.06.017.
33. Monier A, et al. Liver and biliary damages following transarterial chemoembolization of hepatocellular carcinoma: comparison between drug-eluting beads and lipiodol emulsion. Eur Radiol. 2017;27(4):1431–9. https://doi.org/10.1007/s00330-016-4488-y.
34. Guiu B, et al. Liver/biliary injuries following chemoembolisation of endocrine tumours and hepatocellular carcinoma: Lipiodol vs. drug-eluting beads. J Hepatol. 2012;56(3):609–17. https://doi.org/10.1016/j.jhep.2011.09.012.
35. Hong K, Khwaja A, Liapi E, Torbenson MS, Georgiades CS, Geschwind JFH. New intra-arterial drug delivery system for the treatment of liver cancer: preclinical assessment in a rabbit model of liver cancer. Clin Cancer Res. 2006;12(8):2563–7. https://doi.org/10.1158/1078-0432.CCR-05-2225.
36. Wang Q, Hodavance M, Ronald J, Suhocki PV, Kim CY. Minimal risk of biliary tract complications, including hepatic abscess, after transarterial embolization for hepatocellular carcinoma using concentrated antibiotics mixed with particles. Cardiovasc Intervent Radiol. 2018;41(9):1391–8. https://doi.org/10.1007/s00270-018-1989-x.
37. Venkatesan AM, et al. Practice guideline for adult antibiotic prophylaxis during vascular and interventional radiology procedures. J Vasc Interv Radiol.

2010;21(11):1611–30. https://doi.org/10.1016/j.jvir.2010.07.018.
38. Shin JU, et al. A prediction model for liver abscess developing after transarterial chemoembolization in patients with hepatocellular carcinoma. Dig Liver Dis. 2014;46(9):813–7. https://doi.org/10.1016/j.dld.2014.05.003.
39. Woo S, et al. Liver abscess after transarterial chemoembolization in patients with bilioenteric anastomosis: frequency and risk factors. Am J Roentgenol. 2013;200(6):1370–7. https://doi.org/10.2214/AJR.12.9630.
40. Pipa-Muñiz M, et al. The development of early ascites is associated with shorter overall survival in patients with hepatocellular carcinoma treated with drug-eluting embolic chemoembolization. BMC Gastroenterol. 2020;20:1. https://doi.org/10.1186/s12876-020-01307-x.
41. Patel S, Tuite CM, Mondschein JI, Soulen MC. Effectiveness of an aggressive antibiotic regimen for chemoembolization in patients with previous biliary intervention. J Vasc Interv Radiol. 2006;17(12):1931–4. https://doi.org/10.1097/01.RVI.0000244854.79604.C1.
42. Pentecost MJ, Daniels JR, Teitelbaum GP, Stanley P. Hepatic chemoembolization: safety with portal vein thrombosis. J Vasc Interv Radiol. 1993;4(3):347–51. https://doi.org/10.1016/S1051-0443(93)71873-4.
43. Lautin EM, Joshua N, Schoenfel AH, Bakal CW, Haramati N. Radiocontrast-associated renal dysfunction: incidence and risk factors. 1991. [Online]. Available: www.ajronline.org
44. Sohn W, et al. Effect of acute kidney injury on the patients with hepatocellular carcinoma undergoing transarterial chemoembolization. PLoS One. 2020;15:12. https://doi.org/10.1371/journal.pone.0243780.
45. Hussain N, al Otaibi T, Nampoory MRN, Al-Kabeer Hospital M, al Essa H. Saudi Journal of Kidney Diseases and Transplantation contrast media nephropathy: in depth review. 2008. [Online]. Available: http://www.sjkdt.org
46. Francoz C, Durand F, Kahn JA, Genyk YS, Nadim MK. Hepatorenal syndrome. Clin J Am Soc Nephrol. 2019;14(5):774–81. https://doi.org/10.2215/CJN.12451018.
47. Aoe M, et al. Incidence and risk factors of contrast-induced nephropathy after transcatheter arterial chemoembolization in hepatocellular carcinoma. Clin Exp Nephrol. 2019;23(9):1141–6. https://doi.org/10.1007/s10157-019-01751-4.

15 Follow-Up (Response to Treatment, Clinical Management)

Giulio Vallati and Claudio Trobiani

15.1 Response to Treatment

Radiologic response assessment covers a pivotal role for the assessment of treatment success after transarterial chemoembolization (TACE) and has been extensively refined in the past decade [1]. Response to treatment can be evaluated using different criteria such as the World Health Organization (WHO) criteria, the Response Evaluation Criteria in Solid Tumors (RECIST), or the Liver Imaging Reporting and Data System (LI-RADS) assessment score [2–7]. Currently, contrast-enhanced computerized tomography (CT) and magnetic resonance imaging (MRI) play a fundamental role in the management of liver tumors, mostly hepatocellular carcinoma (HCC), and for the evaluation of the therapeutic efficacy of TACE, which is usually monitored and assessed with imaging. This has been linked, also, to the technological advances in imaging modalities and the introduction of new functional imaging [8, 9].

G. Vallati (✉) · C. Trobiani
Department of Radiology, IRCCS Istituto Nazionale Tumori Regina Elena, Rome, Italy
e-mail: giulio.vallati@ifo.it

15.1.1 Imaging Timing and Acquisition Protocol during Follow-Up

As previously mentioned, contrast-enhanced CT and MRI are the most used imaging modalities after locoregional treatments (LRT) of liver lesions, mostly HCC. In head-to-head comparative studies, MRI proved to be the most sensitive and specific modality for the assessment of residual disease following TACE [10]. However, often the employment of the imaging modality of choice is based on a per-institutional protocol, given availability of resources, associated costs, centers' expertise, and patient-related factors (i.e., CT is preferred when ascites is present).

15.1.1.1 Timing

The first monitoring exam after TACE for the evaluation of the oncological response is usually performed at 1 month, 3 months, and then every 3–6 months following treatment, often scheduled by multidisciplinary tumor boards [10]. Other risk-adapted schedules have been suggested in the past but have not gained widespread acceptance [11].

The first assessment at 1 month is crucial since it has been demonstrated that overall survival (OS) has its strongest correlation with an initial response to the treatment (complete and partial response), with patients showing persistent nonresponse in repeated TACE sessions

P. Lucatelli (ed.), *Transarterial Chemoembolization (TACE)*,
https://doi.org/10.1007/978-3-031-36261-3_15

demonstrating a worse prognosis [10]. Indeed, evidence showed that both the initial and the best response predicts OS effectively. However, achievement of treatment response at an early time point is the most robust predictor for favorable outcomes [12].

In 2017, the feasibility of determining whether CT perfusion (CTP) could be useful for evaluating early response after TACE was assessed. Authors showed how CTP parameters were significantly reduced after TACE in responders (PR, CR, $p < 0.001$) while no difference was observed in nonresponders, after 1 day from the procedure, with only 3 out of 21 lesions with complete response recurred and a mean local recurrence-free survival of 19.6 months [13].

15.1.1.2 Imaging Protocols

The most important factor when choosing the imaging modality for monitoring response to treatment is to use the same imaging protocol during the entire patient follow-up (i.e., thin slab to avoid missing small lesions, multiplanar acquisition protocols, administration of the same intravenous contrast media), regardless of the imaging modality per se [14].

For both CT and MRI acquisition of multiple phase—at least dual-phase—imaging is required. The optimal multidetector, multiphasic CT consists of four separate phases: noncontrast, late arterial phase (contrast in the hepatic artery, portal vein, but not in the hepatic veins), portal venous phase (65–85 s from the beginning of injection), and a delayed phase (3–5 min from beginning of injection); MRI timings are the same. However, MRI has other criteria available to assess response to therapy, compared to CT for which the most useful variables are the hyperenhancement in the arterial phase and the contrast washout during the portal and/or delayed phase, just like pretreatment imaging [15]. Indeed, MRI is an imaging modality that allows to assess both morphological and functional criteria. The acquisition protocol for assessment of tumor response to TACE should include T2-weighted imaging both with and without fat suppression, T1-weighted in- and opposed-phase sequences, diffusion-weighted imaging (DWI), and unenhanced followed by dynamic contrast-enhanced (DCE) 3D gradient-recalled echo fat-suppressed imaging using either gadolinium-based extracellular or hepatobiliary agents with subtraction imaging [16, 17]. After standardized image acquisition protocol parameters, it is equally important that image interpretation should be performed by an experienced abdominal radiologist [18].

The best practice envisions the evaluation of tumor response rate to independent blinded multi-readers, according to both m-RECIST and EASL criteria. Also, images interpretation must provide the assessment of nontarget embolization response rate and of new lesions, either into or outside the liver parenchyma [19]

15.1.2 Image Response Evaluation Criteria

In the past, experts realized that conventional bidimensional or unidimensional assessments of the treated lesions did not adequately describe therapeutic effects of interventional therapies (i.e., treatment-induced tumor necrosis does not cause direct and early tumor shrinkage) [2, 20, 21]; the lack of correlation between early lesion changes and correct response assessment led to overtreatment with repeated therapeutic sessions. That is why first in 2002, the WHO with the EASL recommendations and afterward the development of the RECIST criteria v1.0 and 1.1 were defined as standard of reference assessment systems to evaluate tumor response to therapy [22–24], which provide bidimensional measurement of viable (contrast-enhanced) tumor tissue by triphasic imaging. Finally, the modified RECIST (m-RECIST) were developed, providing guidelines to measure the viable part of residual tissue but recommending the unidimensional assessment of the longest viable tumor diameter and the numeric definitions of response according to RECIST [25, 26]. The last refinements of the m-RECIST have been produced in 2020, when novel clarifications and additional recommendation were incorporated in light of emerging challenges in the study and management of HCC [3], by addressing (i) technical guidelines for image acquisition and contrast administration in CT and

MRI; (ii) definition of typical and atypical intrahepatic tumor tissue; (iii) selection, measurement, and assessment of target and nontarget lesions; (iv) combination of viable tumor and overall diameter measurements for global patient assessment; and (v) differentiation of tumor necrosis and viable tumor with reduced perfusion [3]. Both RECIST and m-RECIST provide four response categories: complete response, partial response, stable disease, and progressive disease [27]. The criteria have been particularly successful because they can be easily applied being mostly based on tumor size. The development of these assessment tools was promoted by the acknowledgment that tumor burden is strongly correlated with survival and consequently that monitoring the progression of tumor burden during follow-up imaging studies is considered a valid prediction of OS [28–30]. Also, LI-RADS has been recently proposed as scoring system for assessment of response to therapy [15, 31]. Finally, the Response Evaluation Criteria in Cancer of the Liver (RECICL) developed in 2009 by the Liver Cancer Study Group of Japan, revised in 2015 and in 2021, are worth mentioning. These guidelines were established to provide response evaluation criteria solely devoted to HCC for both clinical practice and clinical trials of HCC treatment, such as molecular-targeted therapies [32–34].

Therefore, as comprehensive overview, size-based classification systems include the WHO criteria (bidimensional) and RECIST (unidimensional), where the size of the treated lesion is measured, regardless of enhancement. Enhancement-based classification systems include EASL (bidimensional), m-RECIST (unidimensional), RECICL, and more recently, LI-RADs (presence or absence of enhancement), where the size of the residual enhancing component is measured for the former two [35].

15.1.2.1 RECIST 1.1: Non-HCC Response Evaluation Criteria

The RECIST 1.1 criteria are used to evaluate tumor response rate in case of liver malignancies, except for hepatocellular carcinoma. Baseline imaging is recommended to be performed within 1 month to treatment initiation, as close as possible to the therapy. The first step is to categorize lesions as measurable or nonmeasurable.

Measurable Hepatic lesions are considered measurable when larger than 10 mm on imaging [4]. Target tissue must be measured in at least one dimension (preferably choosing the plane of the longest measurement). On CT scans, the minimum measurable diameter should be 10 mm. When more than one measurable lesion is present, a maximum of two lesions per organ should be recorded and measured at baseline (altogether five lesions). Although target lesions are usually chosen according to size, it is also important to consider measurement reproducibility: In cases when the largest lesion does not lend itself to reproducible measurement, the next largest lesion that can be measured reproducibly should be selected [36].

Lymph nodes can be considered pathological when larger than 15 mm in short axis, when assessed by CT scan (CT scan slice thickness no greater than 5 mm) [4].

A sum of the diameters (longest for non-nodal lesions, short axis for nodal lesions) for all target lesions will be calculated and reported as the baseline sum diameters.

Nonmeasurable Nonmeasurable lesions are all those that are either <10 mm (organ)/<15 mm (lymph nodes) or truly nonmeasurable (i.e., portal vein thrombosis and ascites). It needs to be specified that lesions localized in areas previously subjected to other LRT are usually not considered measurable unless progressing.

Response Criteria

The evaluation of *target lesions* response to treatment can be categorized in four assessment categories:

- Complete response (CR) can be assigned when disappearance of all target lesions is demonstrated. Any pathological lymph nodes

(whether target or nontarget) short axis should measure less than 10 mm.
- Partial response (PR) will be assigned when there is a decrease of at least 30% in the sum of target lesions' diameters, taking as reference standard the baseline sum diameters.
- Progressive disease (PD) can be demonstrated when patients experience an increase in the sum of diameters of target lesions of at least 20%, taking as reference the smallest sum on study (this includes the baseline sum if that is the smallest on study). Also, regardless of the 20% increase in diameters' sum, a 5 mm increase of the sum itself should be demonstrated, in order to consider the disease as progressive. Finally, the incidence of one or more new lesions is also considered progression.
- Stable disease (SD) can be assigned when there is no sufficient shrinkage to qualify the disease as partially responding or sufficient increase to qualify for progression, taking as reference the smallest sum diameters while on study.

Of note, consider that lymph nodes identified as target lesions should always be measured on their short axis, even if shorter than 10 mm on study. This way, when lymph nodes are included as target lesions, the sum of lesions may not be zero even if complete response criteria are met.

The evaluation of *nontarget lesions* response to treatment can be categorized in three assessment categories:

- Complete response is assigned when there is disappearance of all nontarget lesions and normalization of tumor marker level. All lymph nodes must be non-pathological (<10 mm short axis).
- Non-CR/non-PD can be confirmed when there is persistence of one or more nontarget lesion(s) and/or maintenance of tumor marker level above the normal limits.
- Progressive disease can be assigned when there is an unequivocal progression of existing nontarget lesions or when one or more new lesions are detected [37].

The patient's best *overall response assignment* will be based on the findings of both target and nontarget disease and on the appearance of new lesions. Also, depending on the study itself and the protocol requirements, confirmatory measurement might be also needed to confirm the type of response to therapy; this is needed in nonrandomized trials where response is the primary endpoint of the studies and verification of progression or remission is needed to deem either one of the best overall responses [38, 39].

15.1.2.2 HCC Response Evaluation Criteria (M-RECIST, EASL Criteria, LI-RADS TRA)

Unlike most other solid cancers, conventional chemotherapy has a limited role in patients affected by hepatocellular carcinoma, for which, instead, antiangiogenesis intra-arterial (due to the predominant vascularization of HCC) locoregional therapies are useful therapeutic options [40–42]. These therapies tend to induce tumor tissue necrosis or intratumorally response, not necessarily determining tumor shrinkage. For these reasons, using the WHO criteria and both versions of the RECIST criteria might lead to underestimation of tumor response and consequent overdiagnosis and overtreatment of tumor residues or recurrence [43].

The most important difference of new-generation image response assessment criteria is the concept of "viable tumor," which is strongly related to tumor enhancement [44].

Modified RECIST (m-RECIST) Criteria

M-RECIST is the standard tool for measuring radiological endpoints at early and intermediate stages of HCC, and evidence is growing regarding its relevance in advanced HCC.

The *first step* to apply m-RECIST criteria is to assess tumor lesion at baseline imaging examination and selecting *target lesions:*

- Select intrahepatic tumor lesions ≥1 cm in longest diameter showing intratumorally arterial enhancement and appearing suitable for accurate and repeated measurement. Select *up to two* lesions with these characteristics as *typical intrahepatic target* lesions (defined as lesion that shows intratumoral arterial enhancement on multiphasic contrast-enhanced imaging studies). Additional imaging characteristics such as non-peripheral washout in the portal venous or the delayed phase, or the presence of a capsule, are not required [3].

- In cases where no suitable intrahepatic target lesions are found, it is important to identify lesions ≥ 1 cm in longest diameter, suitable for accurate and repeated measurement even though no intratumoral enhancement is detectable. These will be considered as *atypical target lesions.*
- As already mentioned above, lymph nodes can be considered as extrahepatic target lesions only when the short axis measures >1.5 cm (excluding portal lymph nodes for which the size cutoff for short axis is 2 cm).
- When measuring target lesions, it is crucial to measure the longest viable tumor diameter (excluding internal necrosis areas) or the longest tumor diameter for atypical intrahepatic target lesions or extrahepatic lesions.
- Calculate the baseline sum of target lesions diameters.

In addition, also nontarget lesions should be assessed on baseline imaging:

- Nontarget lesions can be typical or atypical, intrahepatic or extrahepatic lesions. Once a nontarget lesion is described, it is necessary to assess its changes during follow-ups. It is also important to remember that whenever the dominant hepatic lesion is not easily reproducible, it will be categorized as nontarget.
- Any extrahepatic tumor tissue, not classified as target lesions, should be recorded as nontarget (i.e., malignant portal vein thrombosis is the most important). Ascites and pleural effusion cannot be certainly described as tumoral manifestation, so they should not be included in this category.

Once categorization of lesions as target and nontarget is performed, the *next step* for application of the m-RECIST criteria is to *assess tumor response* after treatment on post-procedural imaging studies, by applying the following recommendations:

- *For target lesions*, it is necessary to measure the longest viable tumor diameter of intrahepatic target lesions. Keep in mind that the viable part of the tumor may not be localized on the same slice where the longest tumoral diameter is measured. Areas of necrosis should not be measured. It is crucial, in post-treatment imaging studies, to distinguish between viable tumoral areas and areas of reduced arterial perfusion caused by changes in local hemodynamic mechanisms. A tissue demonstrating a change of vascularization, from hypervascularity to hypovascularity, does not have to be considered tumor necrosis: Only areas that show complete absence of contrast enhancement can be considered necrotic areas.
- For *atypical target lesions,* it is necessary to measure the longest overall tumor diameter, as well as for extrahepatic target lesions.
- Always remember to calculate the sum of diameters of target lesions.
- *For nontarget lesions,* disappearance of enhancement inside malignant portal vein thrombosis should be considered equivalent to complete response.
- *For new lesions,* the appearance of a new liver lesion ≥ 1 cm that shows characteristics of typical lesion determines a progressive disease. Any new liver lesion <1 cm or without typical vascularization pattern can be considered HCC only if it either acquires typical vascularization patterns or shows an interval growth ≥ 1 cm in the follow-up scan.

The *final step* in m-RECIST is treatment response categorization.

- Complete response (CR) is assigned when there is disappearance of any intratumoral arterial enhancement in all typical intrahepatic target lesions AND disappearance of all atypical intrahepatic target lesions and extrahepatic target lesions. Nodal lesions with short axis diameters that regressed to <1 cm can be considered normal.

- Partial response (PR) is assigned the sum of diameters of the target lesions decreases of at least 30% (including viable tumor diameters for typical intrahepatic target lesions and short axis diameters for nodal lesions), taking as reference the baseline sum of the longest diameters.
- Progressive disease is described *when* at least a 20% increase AND an absolute increase of at least 5 mm in the sum of diameters of the target lesions is documented (including viable tumor diameters for typical intrahepatic target lesions and short axis diameters for nodal lesions), taking as reference the nadir sum of diameters recorded since baseline.
- Stable disease is identified when there is not sufficient decrease in size to qualify for PR or sufficient increase of the same to qualify for PD.
- *Not evaluable:* At least one target lesion is not evaluable and the change in the sum of diameters of the measurable target lesions does not meet the criteria for PD.

Overall patient response is a result of the combined assessment of the three categories of target lesions, nontarget lesions, and new lesions. It needs to be kept in mind that evidence of progression in any of these is indicative of overall disease progression; however, the specific progressive category should be clearly reported. While overall disease progression may be captured by isolated progression of nontarget lesions, it must be specified that this is exceptional and that unequivocal findings are required to verify disease progression [3].

Notably, m-RECIST has shown optimal interreader agreement, with values similar or higher compared to those reported for standard RECIST in comparative series [45, 46].

European Association for Study of the Liver (EASL) Response Categories

The EASL criteria use bidimensional measurements and categorize response similarly to the WHO guidelines [22], describing the following response categories:

- Complete response: when there is disappearance of any intratumoral (arterial and portal) enhancement in all target lesion(s) (up to two measurable liver lesions).
- Partial response: when ≥50% decrease in total tumor load (defined as sum of the cross product of two largest diameters or as the sum of surfaces of viable target lesions) of all measurable lesion(s).
- Stable disease when neither PR nor PD can be described.
- Progression disease when more than ≥25% increase in size of one or more measurable lesion(s) or the appearance of new lesion are detected.

Differences Between M-RECIST and EASL

M-RECIST and EASL criteria are both based on measurement of the enhanced lesions, considering the "vial" part of the tumoral node. The main difference is that for the m-RECIST criteria, tumor viability is determined on arterial phase images, and for the EASL criteria, the portal venous phase images can be used as well.

The other difference is that RECIST 1.1 and m-RECIST are criteria based on measuring lesions on a single largest axial diameter and the EASL criteria implies to measure the largest axial bidimensional diameters or the enhanced area of the lesion. This leads to a significant difference in establishing partial response and progressive disease thresholds.

Comparative studies have proved how the EASL criteria proved to underestimate tumor viability and progressive disease compared to RECIST and m-RECIST. Indeed, RECIST criteria demonstrated better accuracy compared with EASL criteria for predicting survival in patients after LT who had transarterial chemoembolization as a "bridge" therapy [47–49].

However, for both m-RECIST and EASL criteria, limitations must be acknowledged: (i) During conventional TACE, an emulsion of a concentrated chemotherapeutic agent and ethiodized oil (Lipiodol, Laboratoire Guerbet,

Villepinte, France) is used. Due to its hyperattenuation on CT, intratumoral Lipiodol deposits can partially mask hyperenhancing portions of tumors, which could lead to overestimation of tumor response after cTACE with m-RECIST [50]. (ii) Concerning nonmeasurable lesions, HCC may present as an ill-defined lesion with infiltrative margins and develop with a predominantly intravascular growth pattern. These forms of the disease are often non-hyperenhanced on arterial phase images. In these cases, m-RECIST and EASL criteria can still be applied to assess tumor response according to RECIST criteria, but the tumor should not be considered as the target lesion [19].

LI-RADS Treatment Response Algorithm

The LI-RADS treatment response algorithm (TRA) was introduced in the 2017 and 2018 updated version of the LI-RADS score and is used to assess HCC after LRT using both CT and MRI [15, 51–53]. According to the recommendations, before scoring imaging using the LI-RADS score, the reader needs to decide whether the treated lesion can be assessed or not based on the presence of suboptimal acquisition protocol and/or the presence of viable tumor.

Therefore, the categorization can be stratified into the following major scores:

- LI-RADS nonevaluable: Image degradation or the omission of necessary enhancement phases does not allow to properly evaluate lesions.
- LI-RADS nonviable: Treated lesions with no enhancement or expected treatment-specific enhancement patterns.
- LI-RADS viable: It can be used to evaluate treated lesions with viable tumor tissue (i.e., enhancing nodular, mass-like, or thick irregular tissue in or along the margin of the treated nodule, with any of the following: arterial phase hyperenhancement (APHE), washout, and enhancement similar to pretreatment enhancement.
- LR-TR equivocal: This category score should be assigned to tumors that are evaluable but that do show equivocal features of viable tumor tissue (i.e., incompletely necrotic tumor and granulation tissue).

To assign a final LI-RADS for treatment response, the readers should perform the following steps: (a) Evaluate whether the lesion is evaluable or not and categorize it according to the definitions described above. (b) Measure viable tumor size by measuring the longest diameter through the enhancing area of the treated lesion but not traversing a nonenhancing area. (c) Perform final check by questioning whether the assigned TR category is reasonable and appropriate.

When compared to other guidelines (i.e., RECIST and m-RECIST), LI-RADS TRA not only provides imaging criteria for the assessment of viable and nonviable tumor tissue, with the introduction of new concepts such as nonevaluable and equivocal, but they also address the variable appearances of tumor tissue after different LRT [31, 54]. Several studies have investigated the performance of LI-RADS TRA in the evaluation of HCC after ablation and have showed promising results [7, 55–57] while at the same time moderate inter-reader reproducibility and no impact on overall survival have been shown [58], different from the m-RECIST [59].

15.1.3 The Role of Quantitative Assessment Tools

Up to date, the assessment of HCC response to treatment after TACE is based on qualitative evaluation of radiologists and is therefore strongly linked to expertise.

A quantitative assessment of tumor heterogeneity is not feasible simply applying international recommendations such as LI-RADS TRA and m-RECIST [60]. That is why in the last years, there is a growing interest in applying AI algorithms and radiomics tools for the assessment of HCC response to therapy, to identify phenotypes by extracting quantitative features from CT and/or MR imaging and for preoperative prediction of treatment response [61–68]. However, the application of these tools in the clinical practice still needs to be implemented, specifically as part of clinical indicator-based predictive nomogram to predict TR in intermediate-advanced HCC and clinical prognosis.

15.1.4 Clinical Management and Conclusion

For all the guidelines, the clinical management of all categories, except for patients showing partial response or progression, imaging should be repeated with the same modality to monitor patient's outcome. Instead, whenever viable tumor and/or increase in size after LRT is detected, according to the criteria used, further management potentially affecting transplantation eligibility are warranted.

To conclude, the use of standardized criteria is strongly recommended for an accurate assessment of response to treatment, since it is both critical and essential for clinical practice and clinical trials.

Also, these guidelines facilitate communication and multidisciplinary care of patients with HCC, a disease for which expertise from several specialties such as diagnostic and interventional radiology, hepatology, transplantation surgery, and surgical, medical, and radiation oncology is required.

References

1. Sieghart W, Hucke F, Peck-Radosavljevic M. Transarterial chemoembolization: modalities, indication, and patient selection. J Hepatol. 2015;62:1187–95. https://doi.org/10.1016/j.jhep.2015.02.010.
2. Therasse P, Arbuck SG, Eisenhauer EA, et al. New guidelines to evaluate the response to treatment in solid Tumors. J Natl Cancer Inst. 2000;92:205–16. https://doi.org/10.1093/jnci/92.3.205.
3. Llovet JM, Lencioni R. mRECIST for HCC: performance and novel refinements. J Hepatol. 2020;72:288–306. https://doi.org/10.1016/j.jhep.2019.09.026.
4. Eisenhauer EA, Therasse P, Bogaerts J, et al. New response evaluation criteria in solid tumours: revised RECIST guideline (version 1.1). Eur J Cancer. 2009;45:228–47. https://doi.org/10.1016/j.ejca.2008.10.026.
5. Schwartz LH, Litière S, de Vries E, et al. RECIST 1.1-Update and clarification: from the RECIST committee. Eur J Cancer. 2016;62:132–7. https://doi.org/10.1016/j.ejca.2016.03.081.
6. Schwartz LH, Seymour L, Litière S, et al. RECIST 1.1—Standardisation and disease-specific adaptations: perspectives from the RECIST Working Group. Eur J Cancer. 2016;62:138–45. https://doi.org/10.1016/j.ejca.2016.03.082.
7. Chaudhry M, McGinty KA, Mervak B, et al. The LI-RADS version 2018 MRI treatment response algorithm: evaluation of ablated hepatocellular carcinoma. Radiology. 2020;294:320–6. https://doi.org/10.1148/radiol.2019191581.
8. Hayano K, Fuentes-Orrego JM, Sahani DV. New approaches for precise response evaluation in hepatocellular carcinoma. World J Gastroenterol. 2014;20:3059–68. https://doi.org/10.3748/wjg.v20.i12.3059.
9. Jiang T, Zhu AX, Sahani DV. Established and novel imaging biomarkers for assessing response to therapy in hepatocellular carcinoma. J Hepatol. 2013;58:169–77. https://doi.org/10.1016/j.jhep.2012.08.022.
10. Kubota K, Hisa N, Nishikawa T, et al. Evaluation of hepatocellular carcinoma after treatment with transcatheter arterial chemoembolization: comparison of Lipiodol-CT, power Doppler sonography, and dynamic MRI. Abdom Imaging. 2001;26:184–90. https://doi.org/10.1007/s002610000139.
11. Boas FE, Do B, Louie JD, et al. Optimal imaging surveillance schedules after liver-directed therapy for hepatocellular carcinoma. J Vasc Interv Radiol. 2015;26:69–73. https://doi.org/10.1016/j.jvir.2014.09.013.
12. Kim BK, Kim SU, Kim KA, et al. Complete response at first chemoembolization is still the most robust predictor for favorable outcome in hepatocellular carcinoma. J Hepatol. 2015;62:1304–10. https://doi.org/10.1016/j.jhep.2015.01.022.
13. Tamandl D, Waneck F, Sieghart W, et al. Early response evaluation using CT-perfusion one day after transarterial chemoembolization for HCC predicts treatment response and long-term disease control. Eur J Radiol. 2017;90:73–80. https://doi.org/10.1016/j.ejrad.2017.02.032.
14. Kloeckner R, Otto G, Biesterfeld S, et al. MDCT versus MRI assessment of tumor response after transarterial chemoembolization for the treatment of hepatocellular carcinoma. Cardiovasc Intervent Radiol. 2010;33:532–40. https://doi.org/10.1007/s00270-009-9728-y.
15. Voizard N, Cerny M, Assad A, et al. Assessment of hepatocellular carcinoma treatment response with LI-RADS: a pictorial review. Insights Imaging. 2019;10:121. https://doi.org/10.1186/s13244-019-0801-z.
16. Braga L, Guller U, Semelka RC. Pre-, Peri-, and Posttreatment imaging of liver lesions. Radiol Clin

N Am. 2005;43:915–27. https://doi.org/10.1016/j.rcl.2005.05.005.
17. Limanond P, Zimmerman P, Raman SS, et al. Interpretation of CT and MRI after radiofrequency ablation of hepatic malignancies. Am J Roentgenol. 2003;181:1635–40. https://doi.org/10.2214/ajr.181.6.1811635.
18. Bouda D, Lagadec M, Alba CG, et al. Imaging review of hepatocellular carcinoma after thermal ablation: the good, the bad, and the ugly: imaging of HCC after thermal ablation. J Magn Reson Imaging. 2016;44:1070–90. https://doi.org/10.1002/jmri.25369.
19. Gregory J, Dioguardi Burgio M, Corrias G, et al. Evaluation of liver tumour response by imaging. JHEP Rep. 2020;2:100100. https://doi.org/10.1016/j.jhepr.2020.100100.
20. Miller AB, Hoogstraten B, Staquet M, Winkler A. Reporting results of cancer treatment. Cancer. 1981;47:207–14. https://doi.org/10.1002/1097-0142(19810101)47:1<207::aid-cncr2820470134>3.0.co;2-6.
21. James K, Eisenhauer E, Christian M, et al. Measuring response in solid Tumors: unidimensional versus Bidimensional measurement. J Natl Cancer Inst. 1999;91:523–8. https://doi.org/10.1093/jnci/91.6.523.
22. Bruix J, Sherman M, Llovet JM, et al. Clinical management of hepatocellular carcinoma. Conclusions of the Barcelona-2000 EASL conference. European Association for the Study of the liver. J Hepatol. 2001;35:421–30. https://doi.org/10.1016/s0168-8278(01)00130-1.
23. Bruix J, Sherman M, Practice Guidelines Committee, American Association for the Study of Liver Diseases. Management of hepatocellular carcinoma. Hepatology. 2005;42:1208–36. https://doi.org/10.1002/hep.20933.
24. Sato Y, Watanabe H, Sone M, et al. Tumor response evaluation criteria for HCC (hepatocellular carcinoma) treated using TACE (transcatheter arterial chemoembolization): RECIST (response evaluation criteria in solid tumors) version 1.1 and mRECIST (modified RECIST): JIVROSG-0602. Ups J Med Sci. 2013;118:16–22. https://doi.org/10.3109/03009734.2012.729104.
25. Lencioni R, Llovet JM. Modified RECIST (mRECIST) assessment for hepatocellular carcinoma. Semin Liver Dis. 2010;30:52–60. https://doi.org/10.1055/s-0030-1247132.
26. Llovet JM, Di Bisceglie AM, Bruix J, et al. Design and endpoints of clinical trials in hepatocellular carcinoma. J Natl Cancer Inst. 2008;100:698–711. https://doi.org/10.1093/jnci/djn134.
27. Gonzalez-Guindalini FD, Botelho MPF, Harmath CB, et al. Assessment of liver tumor response to therapy: role of quantitative imaging. Radiographics. 2013;33:1781–800. https://doi.org/10.1148/rg.336135511.
28. Gillmore R, Stuart S, Kirkwood A, et al. EASL and mRECIST responses are independent prognostic factors for survival in hepatocellular cancer patients treated with transarterial embolization. J Hepatol. 2011;55:1309–16. https://doi.org/10.1016/j.jhep.2011.03.007.
29. Jung ES, Kim JH, Yoon EL, et al. Comparison of the methods for tumor response assessment in patients with hepatocellular carcinoma undergoing transarterial chemoembolization. J Hepatol. 2013;58:1181–7. https://doi.org/10.1016/j.jhep.2013.01.039.
30. Prajapati HJ, Spivey JR, Hanish SI, et al. mRECIST and EASL responses at early time point by contrast-enhanced dynamic MRI predict survival in patients with unresectable hepatocellular carcinoma (HCC) treated by doxorubicin drug-eluting beads transarterial chemoembolization (DEB TACE). Ann Oncol. 2013;24:965–73. https://doi.org/10.1093/annonc/mds605.
31. Kielar A, Fowler KJ, Lewis S, et al. Locoregional therapies for hepatocellular carcinoma and the new LI-RADS treatment response algorithm. Abdom Radiol. 2018;43:218–30. https://doi.org/10.1007/s00261-017-1281-6.
32. Kudo M, Kubo S, Takayasu K, et al. Response evaluation criteria in cancer of the liver (RECICL) proposed by the liver cancer study Group of Japan (2009 revised version). Hepatol Res. 2010;40:686–92. https://doi.org/10.1111/j.1872-034X.2010.00674.x.
33. Kudo M, Ueshima K, Kubo S, et al. Response evaluation criteria in cancer of the liver (RECICL) (2015 revised version). Hepatol Res. 2016;46:3–9. https://doi.org/10.1111/hepr.12542.
34. Kudo M, Ikeda M, Ueshima K, et al. Response evaluation criteria in cancer of the liver version 6 (response evaluation criteria in cancer of the liver 2021 revised version). Hepatol Res. 2022;52:329–36. https://doi.org/10.1111/hepr.13746.
35. Mendiratta-Lala M, Masch WR, Shampain K, et al. MRI assessment of hepatocellular carcinoma after local-regional therapy: a comprehensive review. Radiology: imaging. Cancer. 2020;2:e190024. https://doi.org/10.1148/rycan.2020190024.
36. Schwartz LH, Mazumdar M, Brown W, et al. Variability in response assessment in solid tumors: effect of number of lesions chosen for measurement. Clin Cancer Res. 2003;9:4318–23.
37. Forner A, Ayuso C, Varela M, et al. Evaluation of tumor response after locoregional therapies in hepatocellular carcinoma: are response evaluation criteria in solid tumors reliable? Cancer. 2009;115:616–23. https://doi.org/10.1002/cncr.24050.
38. van Persijn van Meerten EL, Gelderblom H, Bloem JL. RECIST revised: implications for the radiologist. A review article on the modified RECIST guideline. Eur Radiol. 2010;20:1456–67. https://doi.org/10.1007/s00330-009-1685-y.
39. Sargent DJ, Rubinstein L, Schwartz L, et al. Validation of novel imaging methodologies for use as cancer clinical trial end-points. Eur J Cancer. 2009;45:290–9. https://doi.org/10.1016/j.ejca.2008.10.030.

40. Villanueva A. Hepatocellular carcinoma. N Engl J Med. 2019;380:1450–62. https://doi.org/10.1056/NEJMra1713263.
41. Forner A, Gilabert M, Bruix J, Raoul J-L. Treatment of intermediate-stage hepatocellular carcinoma. Nat Rev Clin Oncol. 2014;11:525–35. https://doi.org/10.1038/nrclinonc.2014.122.
42. Tsurusaki M, Murakami T. Surgical and locoregional therapy of HCC: TACE. Liver Cancer. 2015;4:165–75. https://doi.org/10.1159/000367739.
43. Husband JE, Schwartz LH, Spencer J, et al. Evaluation of the response to treatment of solid tumours—a consensus statement of the international cancer imaging society. Br J Cancer. 2004;90:2256–60. https://doi.org/10.1038/sj.bjc.6601843.
44. Arora A, Kumar A. Treatment response evaluation and follow-up in hepatocellular carcinoma. J Clin Exp Hepatol. 2014;4:S126–9. https://doi.org/10.1016/j.jceh.2014.05.005.
45. Tovoli F, Renzulli M, Negrini G, et al. Inter-operator variability and source of errors in tumour response assessment for hepatocellular carcinoma treated with sorafenib. Eur Radiol. 2018;28:3611–20. https://doi.org/10.1007/s00330-018-5393-3.
46. Jeon MY, Lee HW, Kim BK, et al. Reproducibility of European Association for the Study of the Liver criteria and modified response evaluation criteria in solid tumors in patients treated with sorafenib. Liver Int. 2018;38:1655–63. https://doi.org/10.1111/liv.13731.
47. Shuster A, Huynh TJ, Rajan DK, et al. Response Evaluation Criteria in Solid Tumors (RECIST) Criteria are Superior to European Association for Study of the liver (EASL) criteria at 1 month follow-up for predicting long-term survival in patients treated with transarterial chemoembolization before liver transplantation for hepatocellular cancer. J Vasc Interv Radiol. 2013;24:805–12. https://doi.org/10.1016/j.jvir.2013.01.499.
48. Bargellini I, Vignali C, Cioni R, et al. Hepatocellular carcinoma: CT for tumor response after transarterial chemoembolization in patients exceeding Milan Criteria—selection parameter for liver transplantation. Radiology. 2010;255:289–300. https://doi.org/10.1148/radiol.09090927.
49. Haubold J, Reinboldt MP, Wetter A, et al. DSM-TACE of HCC: evaluation of tumor response in patients ineligible for other systemic or loco-regional therapies. Rofo. 2020;192:862–9. https://doi.org/10.1055/a-1111-9955.
50. de Baere T, Arai Y, Lencioni R, et al. Treatment of liver tumors with lipiodol TACE: technical recommendations from experts opinion. Cardiovasc Intervent Radiol. 2016;39:334–43. https://doi.org/10.1007/s00270-015-1208-y.
51. Elsayes KM, Hooker JC, Agrons MM, et al. 2017 version of LI-RADS for CT and MR imaging: an update. Radiographics. 2017;37:1994–2017. https://doi.org/10.1148/rg.2017170098.
52. Gerena M, Molvar C, Masciocchi M, et al. LI-RADS treatment response assessment of combination locoregional therapy for HCC. Abdom Radiol (NY). 2021;46:3634–47. https://doi.org/10.1007/s00261-021-03165-x.
53. Kielar AZ, Chernyak V, Bashir MR, et al. An update for LI-RADS: version 2018. Why so soon after version 2017? J Magn Reson Imaging. 2019;50:1990–1. https://doi.org/10.1002/jmri.26715.
54. Ram R, Kampalath R, Shenoy-Bhangle AS, et al. LI-RADS treatment response lexicon: review, refresh and resolve with emerging data. Abdom Radiol (NY). 2021;46:3549–57. https://doi.org/10.1007/s00261-021-03149-x.
55. Shropshire EL, Chaudhry M, Miller CM, et al. LI-RADS treatment response algorithm: performance and diagnostic accuracy. Radiology. 2019;292:226–34. https://doi.org/10.1148/radiol.2019182135.
56. Do RK, Mendiratta-Lala M. LI-RADS version 2018 treatment response algorithm: the evidence is accumulating. Radiology. 2020;294:327–8. https://doi.org/10.1148/radiol.2020192484.
57. van der Pol CB, Lim CS, Sirlin CB, et al. Accuracy of the liver imaging reporting and data system in computed tomography and magnetic resonance image analysis of hepatocellular carcinoma or overall malignancy—a systematic review. Gastroenterology. 2019;156:976–86. https://doi.org/10.1053/j.gastro.2018.11.020.
58. Pirasteh A, Sorra EA, Marquez H, et al. LI-RADS treatment response algorithm after first-line DEB-TACE: reproducibility and prognostic value at initial post-treatment CT/MRI. Abdom Radiol (NY). 2021;46:3708–16. https://doi.org/10.1007/s00261-021-03043-6.
59. Lencioni R, Montal R, Torres F, et al. Objective response by mRECIST as a predictor and potential surrogate end-point of overall survival in advanced HCC. J Hepatol. 2017;66:1166–72. https://doi.org/10.1016/j.jhep.2017.01.012.
60. Reginelli A, Nardone V, Giacobbe G, et al. Radiomics as a new frontier of imaging for cancer prognosis: a narrative review. Diagnostics (Basel). 2021;11:1796. https://doi.org/10.3390/diagnostics11101796.
61. Kong C, Zhao Z, Chen W, et al. Prediction of tumor response via a pretreatment MRI radiomics-based nomogram in HCC treated with TACE. Eur Radiol. 2021;31:7500–11. https://doi.org/10.1007/s00330-021-07910-0.
62. Guo Z, Zhong N, Xu X, et al. Prediction of hepatocellular carcinoma response to transcatheter arterial chemoembolization: a real-world study based on non-contrast computed tomography radiomics and general image features. J Hepatocell Carcinoma. 2021;8:773–82. https://doi.org/10.2147/JHC.S316117.
63. Svecic A, Mansour R, Tang A, Kadoury S. Prediction of post transarterial chemoembolization MR images of hepatocellular carcinoma using spatio-temporal graph convolutional networks. PLoS One. 2021;16:e0259692. https://doi.org/10.1371/journal.pone.0259692.

64. Dong Z, Lin Y, Lin F, et al. Prediction of early treatment response to initial conventional transarterial chemoembolization therapy for hepatocellular carcinoma by machine-learning model based on computed tomography. J Hepatocell Carcinoma. 2021;8:1473–84. https://doi.org/10.2147/JHC.S334674.
65. Jin Z, Chen L, Zhong B, et al. Machine-learning analysis of contrast-enhanced computed tomography radiomics predicts patients with hepatocellular carcinoma who are unsuitable for initial transarterial chemoembolization monotherapy: a multicenter study. Transl Oncol. 2021;14:101034. https://doi.org/10.1016/j.tranon.2021.101034.
66. Fu S, Chen S, Liang C, et al. Texture analysis of intermediate-advanced hepatocellular carcinoma: prognosis and patients' selection of transcatheter arterial chemoembolization and sorafenib. Oncotarget. 2017;8:37855–65. https://doi.org/10.18632/oncotarget.13675.
67. Zou X, Fan W, Xue M, Li J. Evaluation of the benefits of TACE combined with Sorafenib for hepatocellular carcinoma based on untreatable TACE (unTACEable) progression. Cancer Manag Res. 2021;13:4013–29. https://doi.org/10.2147/CMAR.S304591.
68. Kloth C, Thaiss WM, Kärgel R, et al. Evaluation of texture analysis parameter for response prediction in patients with hepatocellular carcinoma undergoing drug-eluting bead transarterial chemoembolization (DEB-TACE) using biphasic contrast-enhanced CT image data: correlation with liver perfusion CT. Acad Radiol. 2017;24:1352–63. https://doi.org/10.1016/j.acra.2017.05.006.

Miscellaneous 16

Pierleone Lucatelli, Bianca Rocco, Fabrizio Basilico, Stavros Spiliopoulos, Lazaros Reppas, Timo Alexander Auer, Federico Collettini, Marta Burrel, Patricia Bermúdez, Roberto Cianni, Gianluca De Rubeis, Giulio Vallati, Claudio Trobiani, Roberto Iezzi, Rafael Duran, Thierry de Baere, Lambros Tselikas, and Carlo Catalano

P. Lucatelli (✉) · B. Rocco · F. Basilico · C. Catalano
Vascular and Interventional Radiology Unit, Department of Radiological, Oncological, and Anatomo-Pathological Sciences, Sapienza University of Rome, Rome, Italy
e-mail: carlo.catalano@uniroma1.it

S. Spiliopoulos · L. Reppas
2nd Department of Radiology, Interventional Radiology Unit, National and Kapodistrian University of Athens, "ATTIKON" University General Hospital, Athens, Greece
e-mail: stavspiliop@med.uoa.gr

T. A. Auer · F. Collettini
Charitè, Berlino, Germany
e-mail: timo-alexander.auer@charite.de; federico.collettini@charite.de

M. Burrel · P. Bermúdez
Vascular Radiology Unit, Radiology Department, Hospital Clinic, Barcelona Liver Cancer Group (BCLC), Barcelona, Spain
e-mail: MBURREL@clinic.cat; pbermude@clinic.cat

R. Cianni · G. De Rubeis
Dipartimento delle diagnostiche, Azienda Ospedaliera San Camillo Forlanini, Rome, Italy
e-mail: RCianni@scamilloforlanini.rm.it

G. Vallati · C. Trobiani
Department of Radiology, IRCCS Istituto Nazionale Tumori Regina Elena, Rome, Italy
e-mail: giulio.vallati@ifo.it; claudio.trobiani@ifo.it

R. Iezzi
Fondazione Policlinico A Gemelli - IRCCS - Università Cattolica del Sacro Cuore, Rome, Italy

R. Duran
Department of Radiology and Interventional Radiology, Lausanne University Hospital and University of Lausanne, Lausanne, Switzerland
e-mail: rafael.duran@chuv.ch

T. de Baere
Département d'Anesthésie, Chirurgie et Interventionnel (DACI), Gustave Roussy, Villejuif, France

Gustave Roussy Cancer Campus, Université Paris Saclay, Saint-Aubin, France
e-mail: Thierry.DEBAERE@gustaveroussy.fr

L. Tselikas
Département d'Anesthésie, Chirurgie et Interventionnel (DACI), Gustave Roussy, Villejuif, France

Laboratoire de Recherche Translationnelle en Immunothérapie (LRTI), INSERM U1015, Gustave Roussy, Villejuif, France
e-mail: LAMBROS.TSELIKAS@gustaveroussy.fr

P. Lucatelli (ed.), *Transarterial Chemoembolization (TACE)*,
https://doi.org/10.1007/978-3-031-36261-3_16

See Figs. 16.1, 16.2, 16.3, 16.4, 16.5, 16.6, 16.7, 16.8 and 16.9

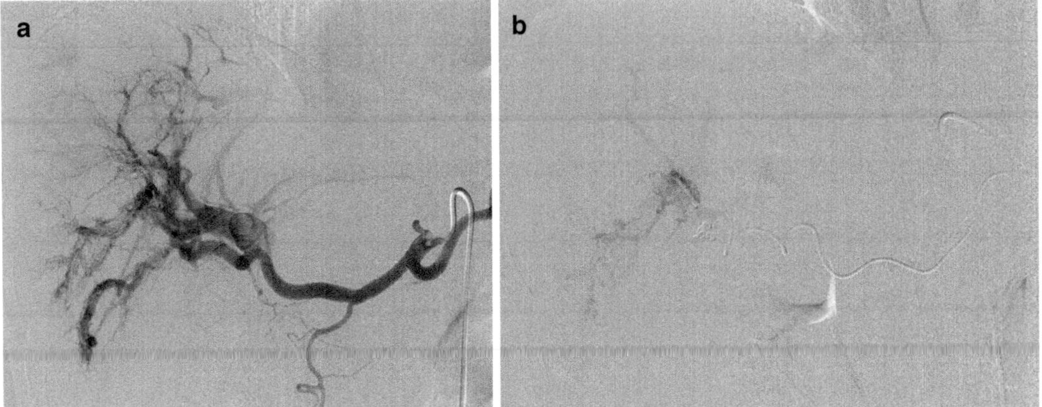

Fig. 16.1 (**a**) Celiac axis DSA depicting a large, high-flow arterioportal communication. (**b**) The communication was embolized using 3 mm pushable micro-coils and DEB-TACE was performed following selective catheterization of the tumor feeding vessel

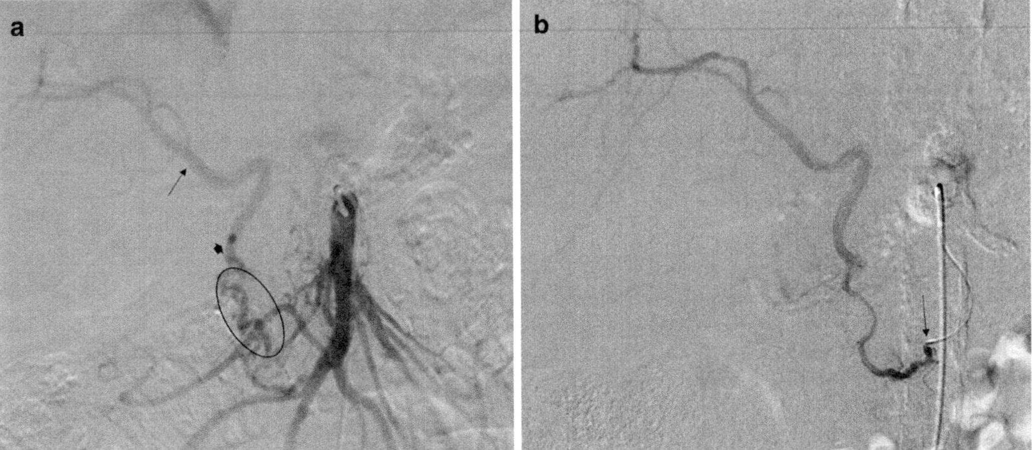

Fig. 16.2 A case of diffuse right lobe HCC and celiac artery occlusion. (**a**) DSA following SMA catheterization depicting the right hepatic artery (arrow) retrogradely perfused via the gastroduodenal artery (arrowhead) and collateral network of the inferior pancreaticoduodenal artery (IPA). (**b**) IPA was selectively catheterized with a microcatheter and DEB-TACE was performed

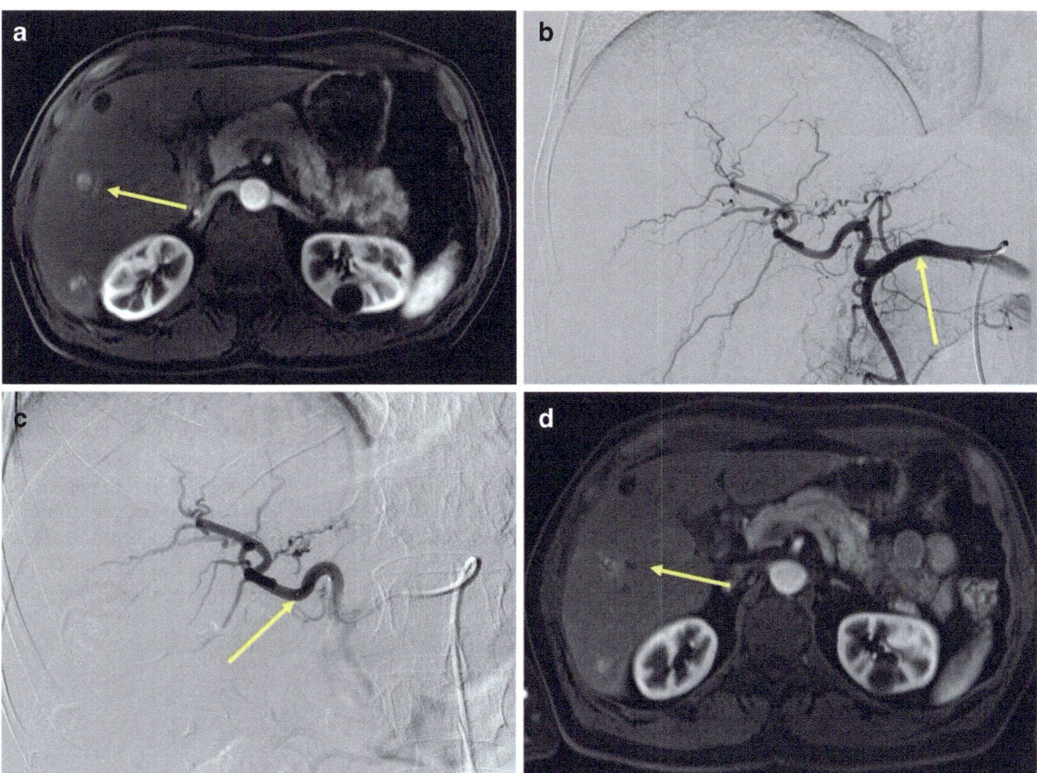

Fig. 16.3 Patient with a multifocal HCC in the right liver lobe treated with DSM-TACE in a lobar fashion. (**a**) Preprocedural MRI (arterial phase) showing two of the multiple hypervascularized HCC lesions in the right liver lobe (yellow arrow, lesion in segment V). (**b**) Celiacography with a 5-F macrocatheter in the main hepatic artery (yellow arrow, tip of the catheter). (**c**) Place of dose application with a 2.5-F microcatheter placed in the proximal right hepatic artery (yellow arrow, tip of the microcatheter). (**d**) Control MRI after 3 months and two sessions of DSM-TACE showing a partial response with partially smaller and devascularized lesions (yellow arrow, lesion in segment V with a reduced lesion diameter and significant devascularization)

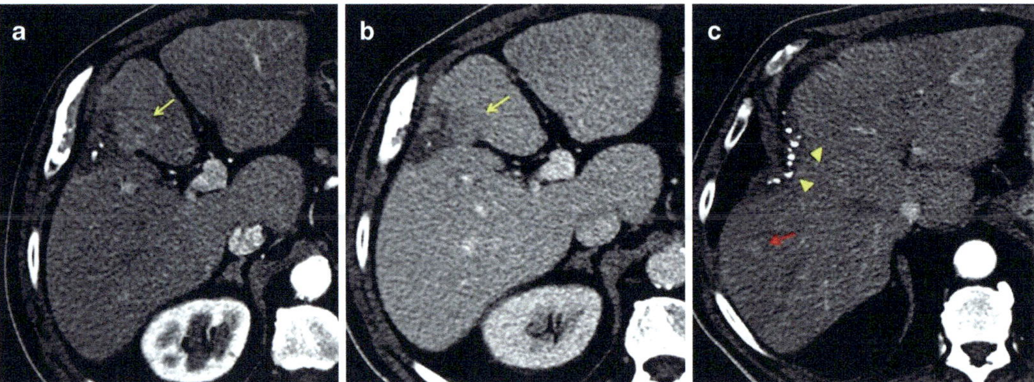

Fig. 16.4 A 73-year-old male with HCV-related cirrhosis, with VII–VIII segmental liver resection for a single HCC, that presents with tumor recurrence 1 year after surgery. CT scan shows viable tumor activity (**a**, **b**, yellow arrows) adjacent to resected area (**c**, yellow arrowheads), and hypervascular infracentimetric nodules nonconclusive of HCC tumors (**c**, red arrow). Selective angiography of the hepatic artery is performed confirming local recurrence (**d**, **e**, **f**) as well as hypervascular infracentimetric nodules (**g**, red arrows). TACE was performed from segmental branches using 100–300 micron DEM, with a total amount of 100 mg of doxorubicin administered, to achieve a complete tumor devascularization (**h**, **i**). The patient presented with postembolization syndrome during admission and mild alteration of ALT/AST that returned to normal within 2 weeks. A follow-up CT scan performed 4 weeks later showed complete tumor response but biliary tract dilatation (**j**, yellow arrows). After recovering from fatigue, a second TACE session was scheduled 3 months later

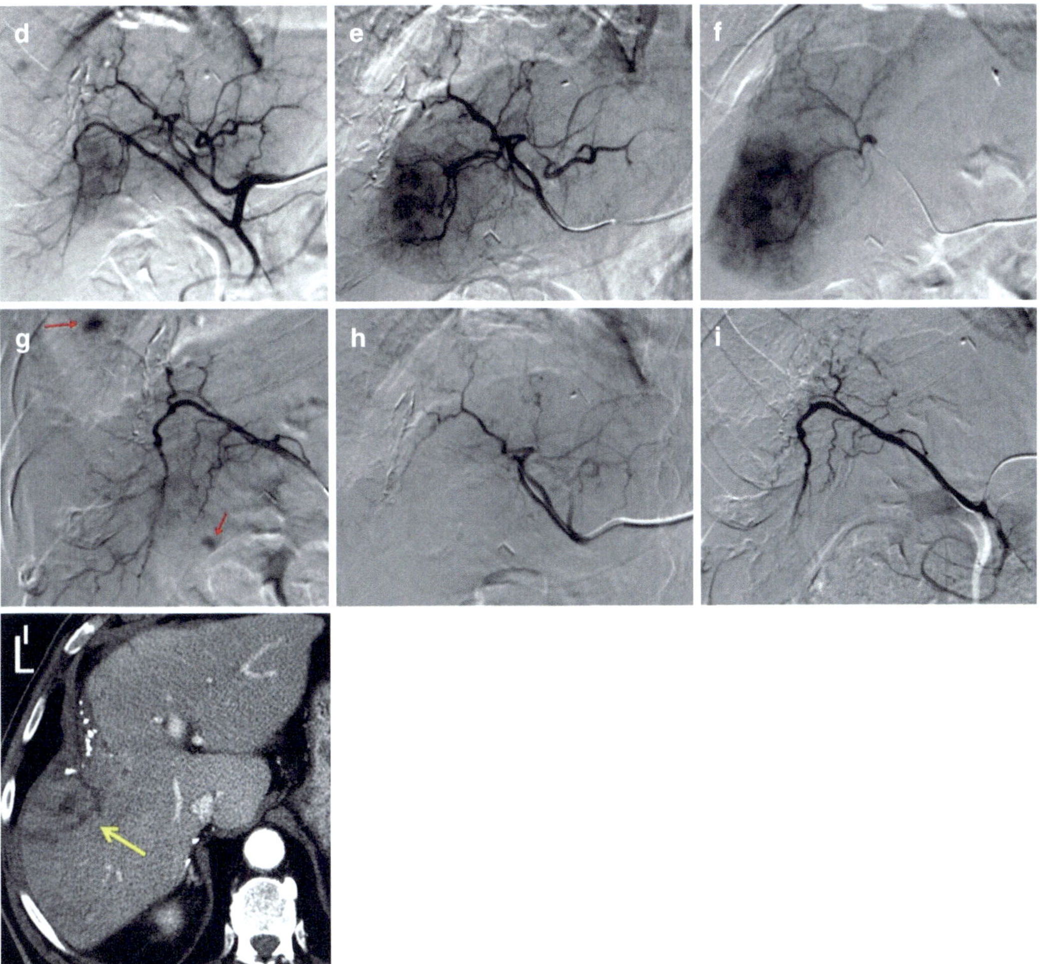

Fig. 16.4 (continued)

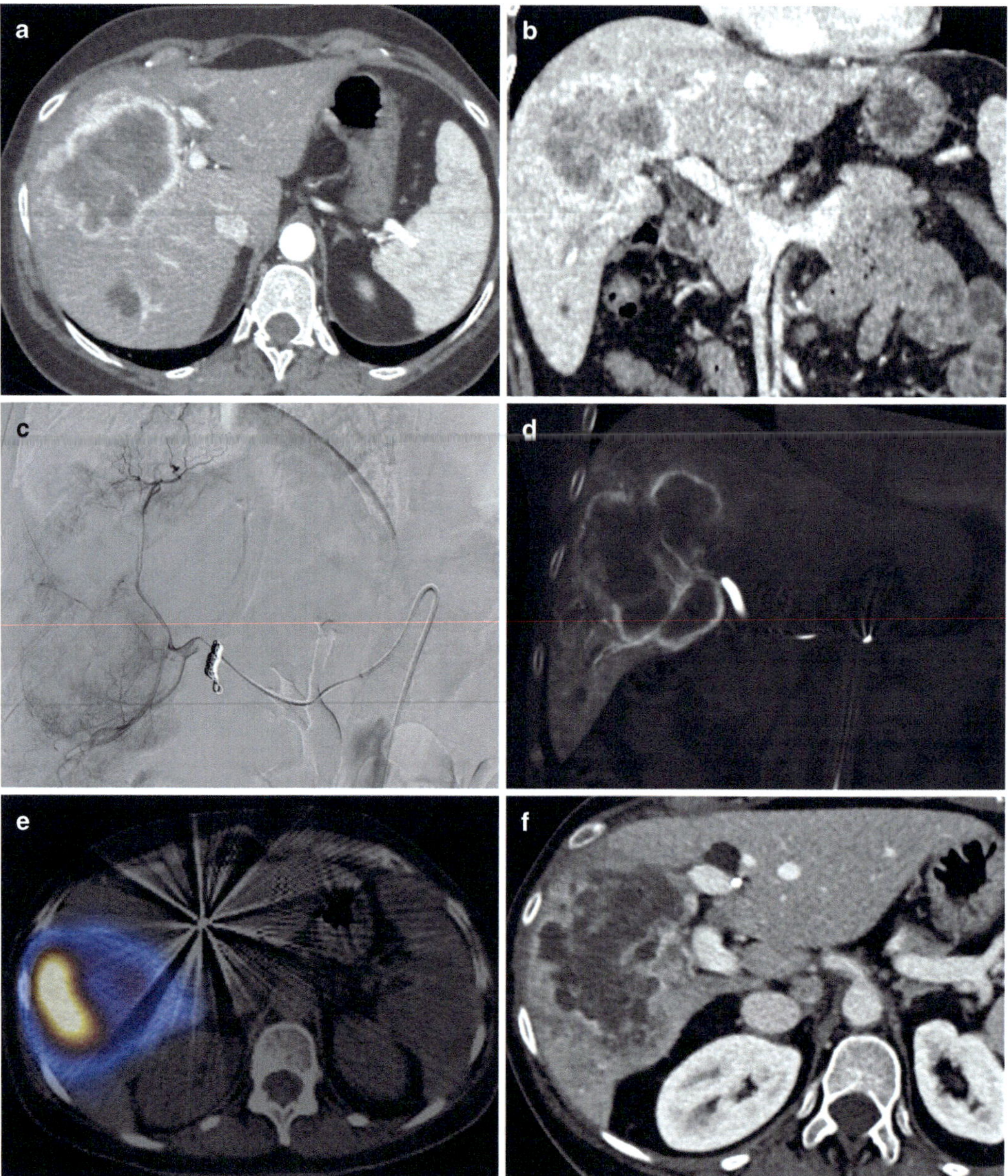

Fig. 16.5 Transarterial radio-embolization (TARE) treatment for intrahepatic cholangiocarcinoma in a 46-year-old woman. Preoperative CT images of a large cholangiocarcinoma in the right hepatic lobe on arterial (**a**) and portal (**b**) phases. Digital subtraction angiography during TARE (**c**), with intra-procedural cone-beam CT scan in arterial phase (**d**). SPECT-CT exam after TARE showing intra-tumoral distribution of Y-90 microspheres (**e**). CT scan performed 1 month after TARE, showing diffuse tumor necrosis (**f**)

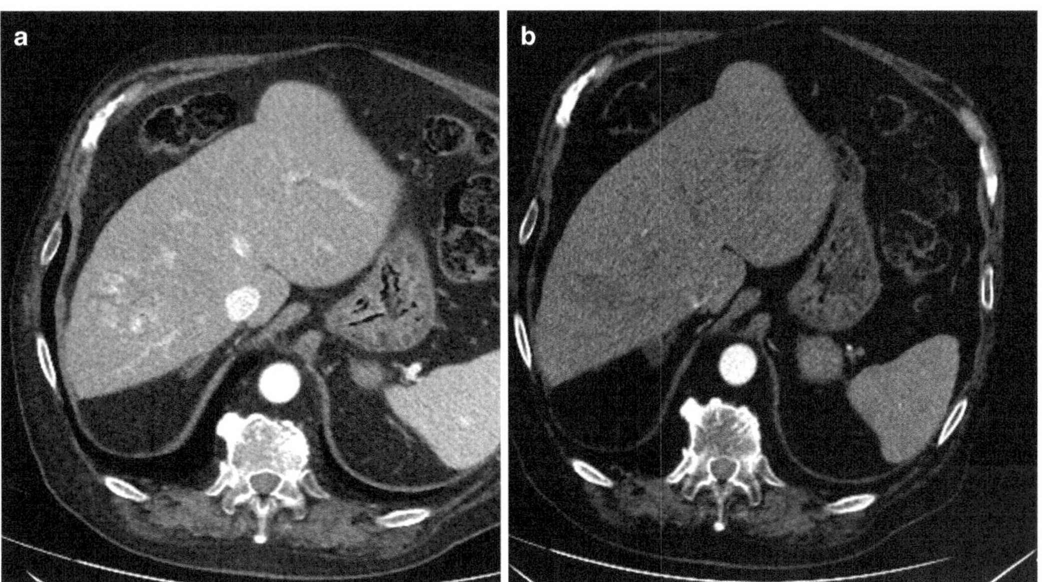

Fig. 16.6 Pretreatment arterial phase CT showing an hypervascular HCC in VII liver segment (**a**). Three months after SIRT arterial phase CT showing disappearance of all hypervascular tumor components configuring a complete response according to mRECIST (**b**)

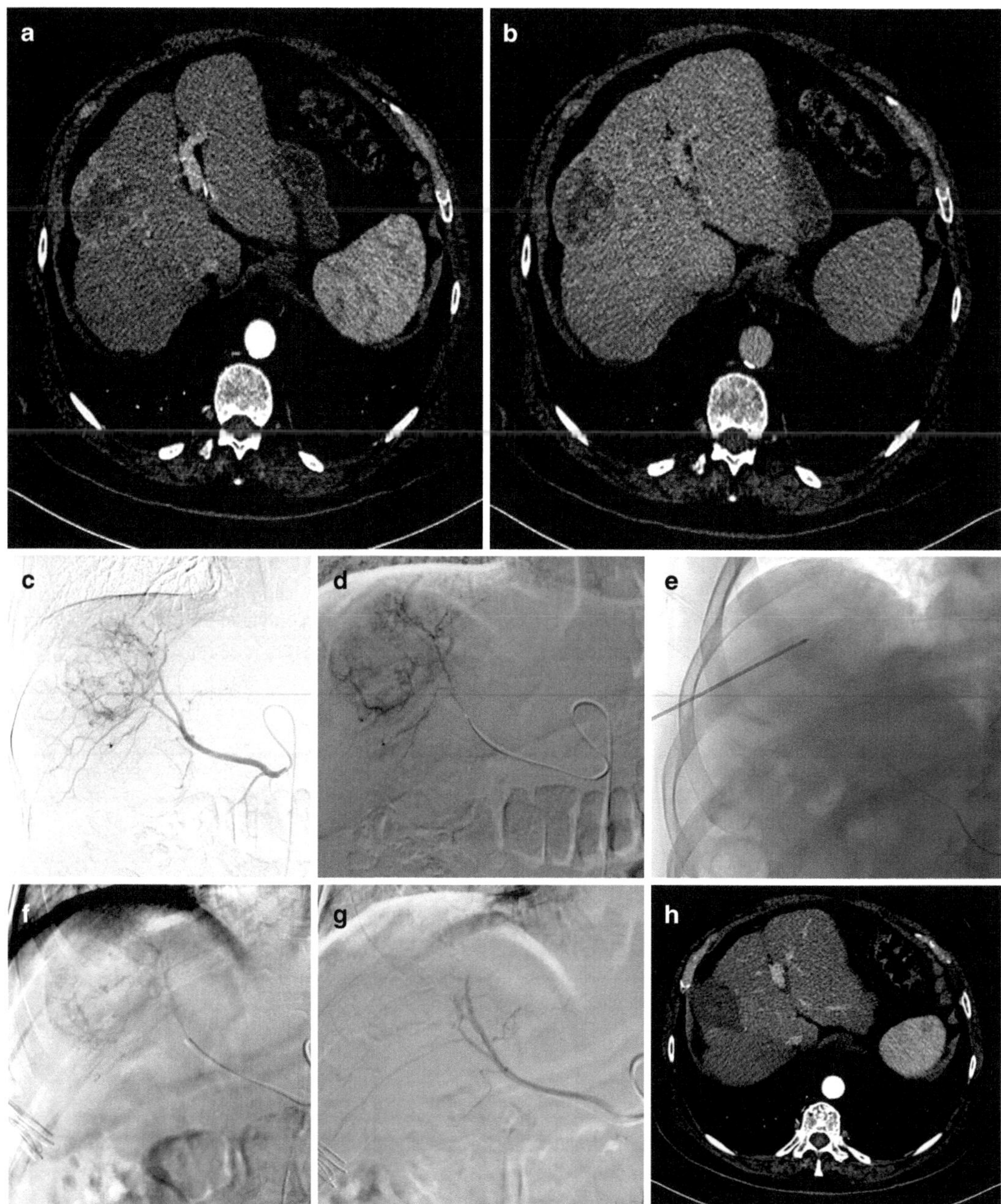

Fig. 16.7 A 79-year-old patient with hepatitis C virus-related hepatic cirrhosis, recent asthenia, weight loss (8 kg), and pancytopenia. Previous asportation of Kaposi sarcoma of the right foot and squamous cell carcinoma of the left eye treated with mitomycin. Baseline CT examination showing a 45 millimeter partly exophytic lesion in the liver segment VIII, with wash-in in the arterial (**a**) phase and washout in the delayed (**b**) phase, respectively, suggestive for HCC (as confirmed by the subsequent liver biopsy). Selective catheterization and angiography of right hepatic artery originating from the superior mesenteric artery confirmed the HCC nodule (**c**). Superselective catheterization of the feeding artery was performed (**d**). Under US guidance, radiofrequency ablation is performed with a 3-cm exposed tip electrode after local anesthesia and during conscious sedation of the patient (**e**). Arteriography performed from the microcatheter in the feeding vessel shows hyperaemia in the target lesion (**f**). Superselective chemoembolization with drug-eluting beads (ranging from 100 to 300 micron) preloaded with 50 mg of doxorubicin is performed until complete dose was administered with complete devascularization of the HCC lesion (**g**). One-month post-procedural CT examination showing complete response to treatment of the target lesion, with complete absence of viable tissue in the arterial phase (**h**)

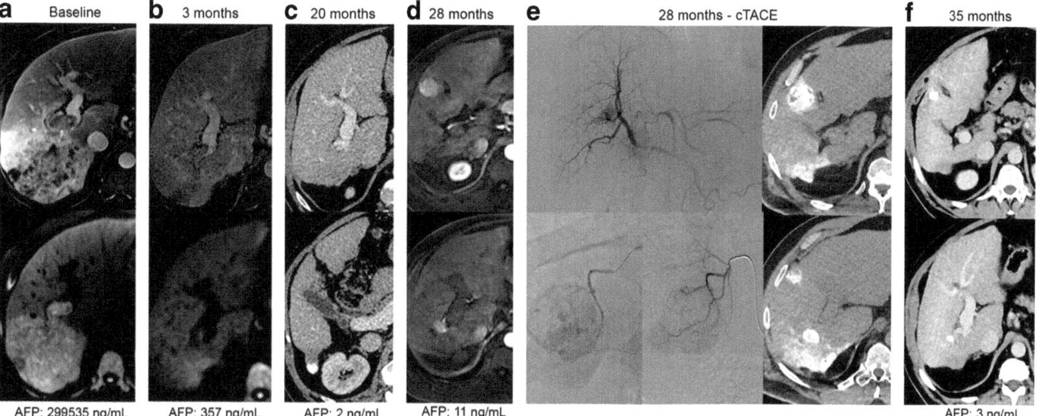

Fig. 16.8 A 62-year-old male with alcoholic cirrhosis (Child-Pugh A) with a 7-cm infiltrative tumor invading the right portal vein consistent with hepatocellular carcinoma (biopsy proven). The patient was given sorafenib but progressed on follow-up MRI with alpha-fetoprotein (AFP) levels of 299,535 ng/mL (**a**). The patient was switched to durvalumab and tremelimumab (Himalaya Trial) with a dramatic response at 3 months on follow-up MRI (**b**). Response still improved and was durable at 20 months from starting the dual checkpoint inhibition (**c**). The patient eventually progressed with the development of a tumor nodule in segment IVB and in the right liver (**d**). The patient was brought to the angiosuite. Celiac trunk angiography shows "tumor blush" of the two nodules (**e**, top). Superselective conventional TACE (c-TACE) was performed in the tumor feeding vessels of these nodules (**e**, bottom). Unenhanced CT performed immediately after c-TACE demonstrates a good uptake of the Lipiodol-based emulsion by the tumors (**e**). Follow-up CT performed at 7 months from c-TACE (35 months from durvalumab and tremelimumab administration) shows a complete response (**f**). This case highlights the potential of combinatorial strategies for liver cancer particularly hepatocellular carcinoma. Courtesy: Gastrointestinal oncology unit at Institut Gustave Roussy

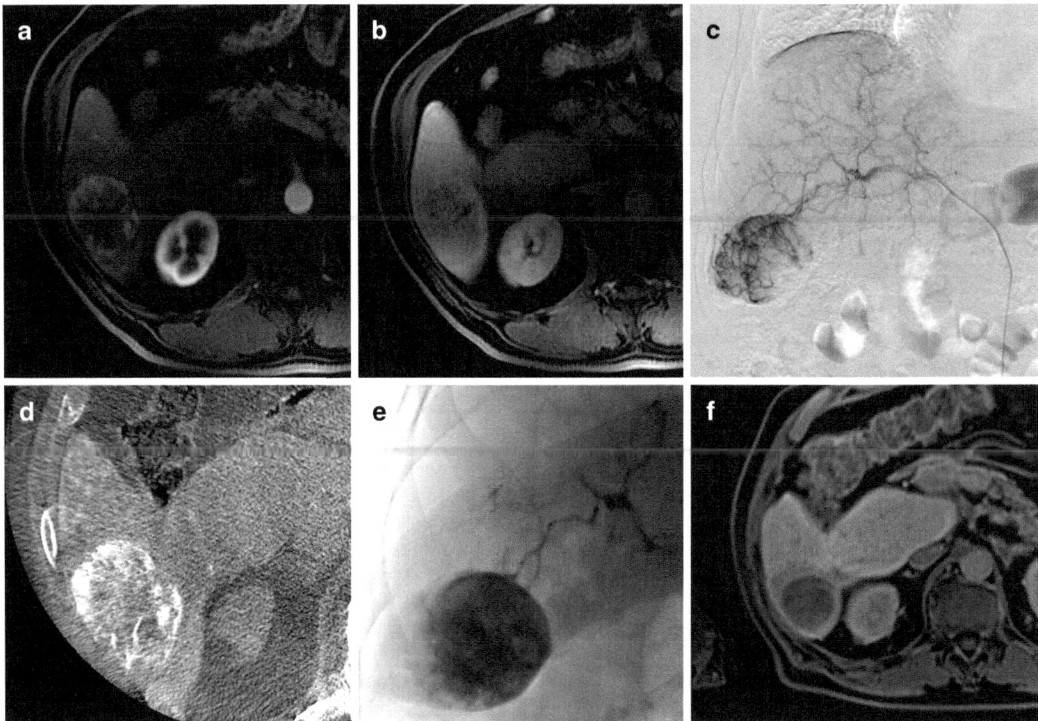

Fig. 16.9 A 61-year-old male with NASH cirrhosis with a 4-cm well-defined and typical HCC (arterial phase CE-MRI (**a**), delayed phase CE-MRI (**b**)) in segment VI confirmed at angiography DSA (**c**) and dual-phase cone-beam CT (**d**) acquired during balloon-occluded TACE procedure. After microballoon inflation, a significative drop of the arterial pressure measured at the tip of the microcatheter was obtained (49 mmHg vs 109 mmHg) and chemoembolization was performed with epirubicin and microspheres (LifePearl, Terumo 100 and 200 micron), with optimal opacification of the tumor (**e**). CE-MRI showed a sustained complete response 3 years after the treatment (**f**)

GPSR Compliance

The European Union's (EU) General Product Safety Regulation (GPSR) is a set of rules that requires consumer products to be safe and our obligations to ensure this.

If you have any concerns about our products, you can contact us on ProductSafety@springernature.com

In case Publisher is established outside the EU, the EU authorized representative is:

Springer Nature Customer Service Center GmbH
Europaplatz 3
69115 Heidelberg, Germany

Batch number: 10371063

Printed by Printforce, the Netherlands